NEW HORIZONS IN LAPAROSCOPIC SURGERY

Edited by **Murat Ferhat Ferhatoglu**

New Horizons in Laparoscopic Surgery
http://dx.doi.org/10.5772/intechopen.69822
Edited by Murat Ferhat Ferhatoglu

Contributors

Alexandre Buckley De Meritens, Adrian Kohut, Leah Goldberg, Jose Pablo Medina, Walter Nardi, Guido Busnelli, Talha Sarigoz, Ozgul Duzgun, Samil Sarici, Mustafa Uygar Kalayci, Paolo Ialongo, Antonio Prestera, Giuseppe Carbotta, Francisco Miguel Sánchez-Margallo, Juan A. Sánchez Margallo, Amir Szold, Tokihito Nishida, Hjime Ikuta, Nidhi Sharma, Vanusha Selvin

First published in London, United Kingdom, 2018 by IntechOpen
IntechOpen is the global imprint of INTECHOPEN LIMITED, registered in England and Wales, registration number: 11086078, The Shard, 25th floor, 32 London Bridge Street
London, SE19SG – United Kingdom
Printed in Croatia

British Library Cataloguing-in-Publication Data
A catalogue record for this book is available from the British Library

Additional hard copies can be obtained from orders@intechopen.com

New Horizons in Laparoscopic Surgery, Edited by Murat Ferhat Ferhatoglu
p. cm.
Print ISBN 978-1-78923-732-0
Online ISBN 978-1-78923-733-7

For EU product safety concerns:
IN TECH d.o.o., Prolaz Marije Krucifikse Kozulić 3, 51000 Rijeka, Croatia,
info@intechopen.com or visit our website at intechopen.com.

Meet the editor

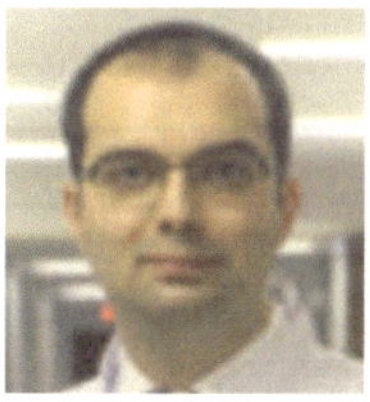

Murat Ferhat Ferhatoglu received his MD degree from the Trace University in Turkey in 2007, and completed his surgical training at the Sisli Etfal Training and Research Hospital in Istanbul in 2014. He served in Bursa State Hospital for three years. Currently, he is an assistant professor at the Okan University, Faculty of Medicine. He has published many articles and holds membership with fellowship of the Turkish Board of Surgery.

Contents

Preface

The first laparoscopic cholecystectomy was performed by French surgeon Mouret in 1987, and this surgery is considered to be the beginning of a video-laparoscopic surgery. What is not to be confused here is that this is not the beginning of a laparoscopic surgery, but the beginning of a video-laparoscopic surgery. The first diagnostic laparoscopy was performed at the beginning of the twentieth century; the first surgical laparoscopy started in the third decade of the twentieth century. After 1950, laparoscopic surgery has entered into a faster development and spreading process, thanks to improvements in lens and light systems, and has been widely used not only for diagnostic purposes but also for therapeutic purposes. Laparoscopic surgery was more commonly used by gynecologists, and the first laparoscopic appendectomy was performed by Kurt Sem, a gynecologist, in 1982. Thanks to the discovery of microprocessors in the 1980s, the dimensions of the camera and light systems have become very small, and laparoscopic surgery has become more common in daily practice. Dr. Mouret's first laparoscopic cholecystectomy operation in 1987 was considered a sensational event and was the beginning of today's modern laparoscopic surgery. In this book, we intend to introduce some new surgical techniques to readers. I would like to thank all the authors who contributed to the preparation of this book.

M.D. Murat Ferhat Ferhatoglu
Okan University
Faculty of Medicine
Department of Surgery
Istanbul, Turkey

Section 1

Surgical Procedures

Chapter 1

Laparoscopic Appendectomy

Paolo Ialongo, Giuseppe Carbotta and
Antonio Prestera

Additional information is available at the end of the chapter

http://dx.doi.org/10.5772/intechopen.74192

Abstract

Appendectomy represents a fundamental step in the training course of a surgeon in so much that for several decades it has been the first surgical operation assigned to a training surgeon. Yet, laparoscopic appendectomy has not spread with the same characteristics as the operation of cholecystectomy for which laparoscopy has rapidly become the gold standard. We can moreover note that nowadays, in spite of a certain initial distrust, the laparoscopic methodology is fully employed in the treatment of acute appendicitis, even though the use of such technique is controversial in cases of acute complicated appendicitis.

Keywords: appendicitis, surgery, laparoscopy

1. Introduction

Appendectomy represents a fundamental step in the training course of a surgeon in so much that for several decades it has been the first surgical operation assigned to a training surgeon.

Yet, laparoscopic appendectomy has not spread with the same characteristics as the operation of cholecystectomy for which laparoscopy has rapidly become the gold standard.

In fact, before attempting their laparoscopic appendectomies, many surgeons have, first, standardised their technique of cholecystectomy. There are many reasons that justify a slower spreading of this methodology:

- Open appendectomy has been considered for decades as a rapid technical method requiring a small surgical incision.

- The operation is, moreover, generally made on an organ suffering from an inflammatory process which often causes a pathological alteration of the surrounding organs with formation of oedema, congestion and adhesions, thus making a laparoscopic appendectomy more difficult.

The open appendectomy introduced by an American surgeon Charles McBurney in 1894 is still today considered the gold standard in the surgical treatment of acute appendicitis because it is a safe surgical procedure, with a low morbidity rate, a short hospitalisation and a low discomfort for the patients. Expected intraoperative difficulties in laparoscopic appendectomy could be the management of peritonitis grade and of ectopic appendix.

The first video-assisted appendectomy seems to have been performed in 1977 by the Dutchman Hans J. De Kok, whose priority is actually unknown owing to the scanty circulation of the medical review which was published.

It was Kurt Semm, a German gynaecologist, who publicised the technique of a laparoscopic appendectomy in his two successive works (June 1982 and January 1983). Semm did not however consider the laparoscopic procedure fit for the case of acute appendicitis, as he confirmed in one of his articles published on the review "Endoscopy" in 1983. But he did not quote any personal case history or experience, thus exposing himself to much criticism.

Actually, in 1987 his countryman Jorg H. Schreiber, from Dusseldorf, published his first dense report of 70 cases in 5 years (of which 67 are made with the laparoscopic technique; 7 with a clinical picture of acute, catarrhal or phlegmonous appendicitis), claiming that he had performed his first laparoscopic appendectomy in June 1982.

The number of publications has been in constant growth since then, and more and more numerous perspective comparative studies show the validity and the safety of the laparoscopic procedure offering such significant advantages as fewer infections of the wound, reduced administration of analgesics and a faster return to normal activity, whereas some authors report that costs are increased and operative time are supposed to be longer than the open procedure.

We can moreover note that nowadays, in spite of a certain initial distrust, the laparoscopic methodology is fully employed in the treatment of acute appendicitis, even though the use of such technique is controversial in cases of acute complicated appendicitis.

Notwithstanding, of the numerous studies that have been published on this subject, there is not yet scientific evidence of the superiority of the laparoscopic technique [1] over the open surgical operation even though the laparoscopic procedure proves to be safe also in complicated case with diffuse peritonitis; in which cases it also allows to perform an accurate lavage of the abdominal cavity.

Despite each patient needs to be evaluated for the best surgical procedure, there is no absolute contraindication to laparoscopic appendectomy in cases of complicated appendicitis, especially for experienced surgeons, because it has been demonstrated that the patients in those cases gain a better postoperative outcome.

Open appendectomy presents a higher incidence of complications (wound infections, which can cause longer hospitalisation) and later postoperative hernias.

Laparoscopic procedure can assure a complete exploration of abdominal cavity, without a bigger incision and in case of ectopic or complicated appendicitis. In those cases, if conversion is needed, it could be possible that a focused incision can be practised. Mini-invasive technique is also useful to treat other associated diseases (previously referred or diagnosed during the surgery).

Among all advantages, described in literature, we must remember the reduction of wound infection incidence, of adhesion-related disorders (very important in young women because of infertility that can be caused by adhesions post appendicitis or salpingitis) and of postoperative pain, a faster hospitalisation, a quick return to daily activity and good aesthetic results.

For all these reasons, laparoscopic appendectomy seems to be destined to become unanimously the gold standard for the treatment of acute complicated appendectomy, just as it happened to laparoscopic cholecystectomy.

2. Epidemiology

Acute appendicitis manifests itself at all ages, mostly during infancy and adolescence; it mainly interests the male sex and has an annual incidence of 0.2%. About 14% of the population is estimated to get acute appendicitis during their lifetime. An early diagnosis and its urgent surgical operation are fundamentals to prevent complications and morbidity.

3. Indications

The advantages of a mini-invasive approach evidence themselves above all among women in childbearing age in whom the differential diagnosis is greatly improved. In this way the diagnosis of such pelvic pathologies which may fake an appendicitis as endometriosis, salpingitis and complications of ovarian cysts like torsions or ruptures of haemorrhagic corpus luteum is made possible, thus reducing the percentage of "innocent" appendicitis, as important meta-analyses clearly show [2]. The diagnostic advantage among children and members of the male sex seems to be less, since in this subgroup of patients the diagnosis of appendicitis and the probable differential diagnosis are simpler; anyway, a considerable percentage of cases (5.5%) is recorded where the diagnosis is modified and corrected by resorting to the laparoscopic technique [2]. In obese patients the postoperative complications of a laparoscopic appendectomy are fewer than those with an open technique. The laparoscopic methodology is applicable also to elderly patients, subject to preoperative diagnosis and in the absence of side effects in general. In literature there seems to be some advantage in favour of laparoscopic appendectomy; a more accurate preoperative diagnostic workup is anyway advised in consideration also of the greater incidence of neoplasias among elderly people [1, 3, 4]. There is no unanimous agreement about laparoscopic appendectomy on pregnant women. The most recent studies on this topic, though they consider the second 3 months as the safest period, do not warn against it during the other periods. Anyway, considering the relative benefits, as well as the potential risks (increase of mortality of foetuses), basing on the data recorded in literature, it is not advisable to prefer laparoscopic appendectomy during all the 3 months of pregnancy [1, 5, 6]. If at the laparoscopic exploration the appendix is shown to be macroscopically undamaged and another pathology is found out as the cause of the symptomatology, there is sufficient evidence that the appendix should not be removed. The difference is the case in which the appendix is normal, but no other pathology is found out; concerning this, it is worthwhile remembering the objective at difficulty, in some cases, of performing a macroscopic diagnosis of appendicitis. In fact an appendix under an initial inflammatory process may have a normal aspect but may result pathologically in the final histological examination. In such cases the surgeon shall decide case by case, on the basis of the preoperative clinical picture. The greater number of authors is in favour of exeresis, also in consideration of the improvement of the clinic symptomatology of such cases. In case of a complicated appendicitis, resorting to the laparoscopic approach is a questionable matter. According to the data recorded in literature, laparoscopy is feasible with the same amount of morbidity as with open technique, in spite of the increase of the incidence of intra-abdominal abscesses which are, on the other hand, counterbalanced by a minor incidence of infections of the wound. The greater incidence of postoperative abscesses may depend either on the relative inexperience of the surgeon or on defects in the surgical technique. The postoperative outcome in terms of total morbidity, hospitalisation and return to work seems, however, to be significantly better among patients with complicated appendicitis treated with the laparoscopic technique. As a matter of principle, the presence of peritonitis, of an abscess, of a gangrenous appendicitis or of perforation does not represent an indication to conversion to laparotomy. Each case must be judged separately, on the basis of the surgical and laparoscopic experience of the surgeon. Conversion to laparotomy is, however, advisable; any time the surgeon does not consider it safe to carry on the surgical operation by laparoscopy, and in such cases, it appears reasonable to make use of an access sufficiently large as to allow to explore and wash the abdominal cavity in an adequate way [7–10].

4. Surgical technique

4.1. Position of the patient

The patient is laid on his back on the surgical bed, with joined and blocked limbs. The right arm is extended laterally (abduction at 90°) so as to allow the anaesthetist's easy vascular access as well as the checking of the vital parameters; the left arm, completely abducted, is fixed to the body. During the surgical operation, some changes of position may be necessary (Trendelenburg, anti-Trendelenburg, left or right lateral inclination) which imply a good anchorage of the patient to the operative table, as accurately as the gravity of the clinical picture requires. In case of serious peritonitis, in fact, washing of the peritoneal cavity is made easier by varying the position of the patient.

4.2. Positioning of the team

The surgical team is made up of the surgeon, the assistant and the instrumentalist operator. This one must stand on the left side of the patient with the surgeon on his right, while the assistant, initially on the right of the patient, shall also move to the left between the surgeon and the instrument operator, after the insertion of the trocars. The service table is laid on the feet of the patient, on the left of the instrumentalist operator.

4.3. Positioning of the trocars

Umbilical, above pubis and in the left iliac fossa are considered the best ports so as to permit an optimal triangulation (**Figure 1**).

The Italian surgical school unanimously favours the technique of three trocars centred in the left hemi-abdomen as described in the early 1990s. The strong points of this position are the easiness of vision and of triangulation, but there is no evidence in literature of an improvement

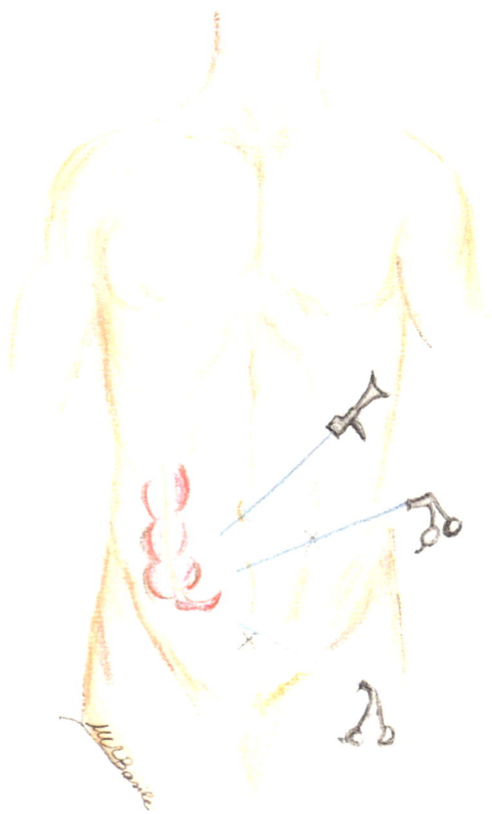

Figure 1. Positioning of the trocars.

of the outcome in comparison with other laparoscopic ports. The insertion of the second trocar in the region above pubis can sometimes present some difficulties; the parietal peritoneum may in fact easily come off the muscle planes, so the needle of the trocar does not pierce it completely but carries it into the abdominal cavity. It is therefore advisable while controlling the manoeuvre through the optical device on the first trocar to carry out the positioning of the trocar in the left iliac fossa as second positioning and not as third positioning; through the iliac trocar, a tenaculum can be introduced so as to press the parietal peritoneum outwards, thus facilitating its penetration. Some surgeons prefer to place the bladder catheter before introducing the trocar above the pubis region to empty the bladder to avoid iatrogenic damages. The use of the two trocars has been studied retrospectively, without evidencing significant advantages. The "single-port" technique has been described in some studies that have shown reduction of the surgical trauma, of the pain and of the postoperative stay in bed, as well as better aesthetic results, but there are still few evidences that it can be an adequate alternative to the standard laparoscopic technique, just as it is the case both with the micro-laparoscopic technique and with the NOTE technique (natural translumenal endoscopic surgery) which makes use of the transvaginal port.

4.4. Exploration of the abdominal cavity

As usual, in all surgical operations either laparoscopic or open, at the start, a careful exploration of the abdominal cavity is necessary with the aim of confirming the diagnosis and/or evidencing other problems. Then, with two atraumatic tenacula (Johanne type), the appendix is searched for by locating the caecum and then the terminal iliac loop. Sometimes, the appendix may take an unusual position (back to the caecum, go down into the Douglas cavity or be adherent to the abdominal wall). In such cases its finding may result difficult. Once the appendix is located, it must be isolated from possible inflammatory-type adhesions.

4.5. Coagulation and section of the meso-appendix

We take note of the great variety of possible usable devices, and we consider bipolar coagulation of the preferable method for the section of the meso-appendix because it is safer and cost-effective (**Figure 2**), even though more rapid, efficient and even more costly methods (e.g. ultrasounds) have been the subject of studies in literature. The appendix is tightened by means of Johanne-type tenacula, and with the chosen device, the meso-appendix is coagulated, starting from the free side towards the appendicular base. Much attention must be paid close to the appendicular artery which must be tied up and sectioned (either directly by means of electricity or by using two clips).

4.6. Tying up the appendicular base

The appendicular stump is closed up by positioning the loop (**Figure 3**), following the methodology already described by Semm in 1983; the mechanical endoscopic stitcher, the stapler, is an alternative approach much employed recently. When using loops, two of them are placed at the base, a few millimetres one from the other. When the stapler is employed, it must comprise the base of the appendix with a piece of caecum as large as a stamp to ensure safe

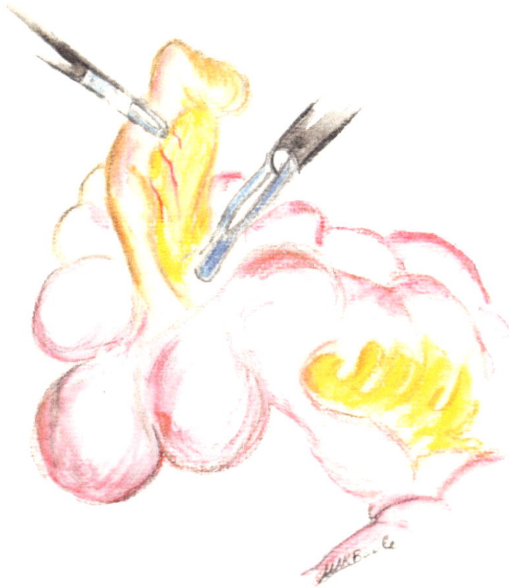

Figure 2. Coagulation and section of the meso-appendix.

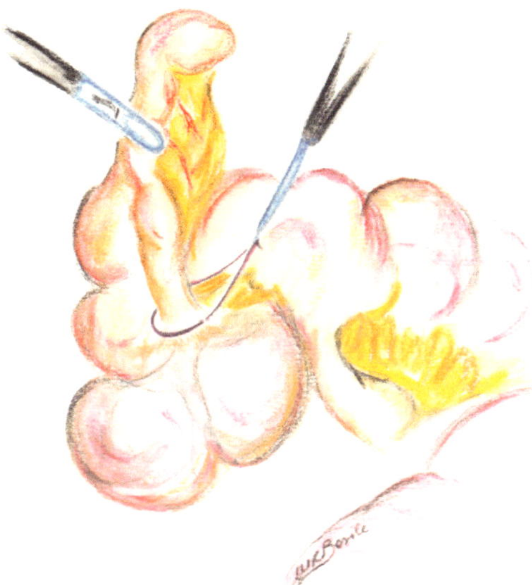

Figure 3. Tying up of the appendicular base.

closure. Numerous comparative studies have been published about these two approaches. Those in favour of the use of a stapler underline such advantages of this technique as the possibility of using it even in complicated appendicitis, reduction of the operating time and of the formation of endo-abdominal abscesses and a fast post-operation canalization of faeces not to mention the easy use on the part of training surgeons. The authors in favour of the use of loops point out an unmeaningful difference between the two techniques, except for the operating time. The looping technique is considered also a good exercise of manual skill for young surgeons and an economic aid, differently from the stapler which, for the same reason, is not economic for a systematic use [1, 11]. The disadvantages of using the loop are, instead, represented by the large learning curve as well as by its not-yet-clear role in complicated appendicitis [1]. In sectioning the viscera, an adequate length of the residual stump is recommended, which inside must be free of coprolites. Appendicitis of the stump is a rare entity but much attention must be paid to the remaining part of the appendix to minimise such a complication [12]. To further reduce costs, some authors advise to make use of reabsorbing clips (hem-o-lok) to suture the appendix but only in the catarrhal forms.

4.7. Removal of the appendix

It is recommended in all cases to protect the abdominal wall accurately during the extraction of the viscera, either by means of endo-bags, by extraction within the trocar or by other aids which may avoid contamination. Infections of wound are remarkably reduced with the laparoscopic appendectomy thanks to the routine use of protection of the operating piece during the extraction. In those cases in which protection is not employed (e.g., in the so-called laparo-assisted one trocar technique), the incidence of postoperative infections rises up to levels which can be compared to those of the open technique [13]. In case of widespread peritonitis, abscess or perforated appendix, a complete peritoneal washing is recommended. The fact of finding postoperative intra-abdominal abscesses in noncomplicated appendix laparoscopically treated has raised the doubt that limited and aimed washing may reduce the incidence, even if only one retrospective study supports this hypothesis [14, 15]. Therefore, in cases of localised phlogosis, aspiration of the effusions by means of localised washing is considered a protective measure against spreading the septic content towards the recesses unharmed by phlogosis. The routine use of drainage is not advisable; it can, however, be useful for therapeutic purposes either in the presence of abscess cavity and of widespread peritonitis [16] or for preventive treatment in particular situations of risk (steroidal therapy, chronic pathologies) and in special patients. In the other cases, the use of drainage is not necessary and can even be harmful.

Author details

Paolo Ialongo[1]*, Giuseppe Carbotta[1] and Antonio Prestera[1,2]

*Address all correspondence to: ialongopaolo@gmail.com

1 General Surgery Unit, Department of Emergency and Organ Transplantation, School of Medicine, "Aldo Moro", University of Bari, Bari, Italy

2 Surgery Unit, Hospital of Gallipoli, Lecce, Italy

References

[1] Gorter RR, Heij HA, Eker HH, Kazemier G. Laparoscopic appendectomy: State of the art. Tailored approach to the application of laparoscopic appendectomy? Best Practice & Research. Clinical Gastroenterology. February 2014;**28**(1):211-224

[2] Tzvoras G, Liakou P, Baloyiannis I, et al. Laparoscopic appendectomy: Differences between male and female patients with suspected acute appendicitis. World Journal of Surgery. 2007;**31**:409-413

[3] Baek HN, Jung YH, Hwang YH. Laparoscopic versus open appendectomy for appendicitis in elderly patient. Journal of the Korean Society of Coloproctology. 2011;**27**(5):241-245

[4] Kirshtein B, Perry ZH, Mizrahi S, Lantsberg L. Value of laparoscopic appendectomy in the elderly patient. World Journal of Surgery. 2009;**33**:918-922

[5] Jackson H, Granger S, Price R, et al. Diagnosis and laparoscopic treatment of surgical diseases during pregnancy: An evidence -based review. Surgical Endoscopy. 2008; **22**:1917-1927

[6] Walsh CA, Tang T, Walsh SR. Laparoscopic versus open appendectomy in pregnancy: A systematic review. International Journal of Surgery. 2008;**6**:339-344

[7] Ferranti et al. Laparoscopic versus open appendectomy for the treatment of complicated appendicitis. Il Giornale di Chirurgia. 2012;**33**(8/9):263-267

[8] Lim SG, Jung Ahn E, Kim SY, Il YC, Park J-M, Choi S hY PKW. A clinical comparison of laparoscopic versus open appendectomy for complicated appendicitis. Journal of the Korean Society of Coloproctology. 2011;**27**(6):293-297

[9] Yau KK, Siu WT, Tang CN, et al. Laparoscopic versus open appendectomy for complicated appendicitis. Journal of the American College of Surgeons. 2007;**205**:60-65

[10] Cueto J, D'Allemagne B, Vazquez-Frias JA, et al. Morbidity of laparoscopic surgery for complicated appendicitis: An international study. Surgical Endoscopy. 2006;**20**:717-720

[11] Sajid MS, Rimple J, Cheek E, Baig MK. Uso of endo-GIA versus endo-loop for securing the appendicular stump in laparoscopic appendectomy: A systematic review. Surgical Laparoscopy, Endoscopy & Percutaneous Techniques. 2009;**19**:11-15

[12] Truty MJ, Stulak JM, Utter PA, et al. Appendicitis after appendectomy. Archives of Surgery. 2008;**143**:413-415

[13] Romy S, Eisering MC, Bettschart V, et al. Laparoscope use and surgical site infections in digestive surgery. Annals of Surgery. 2008;**247**:627-632

[14] Gupta R, Sample C, Barnehriz F, Birch DW. Infectious complications following laparoscopic appendectomy. Canadian Journal of Surgery. 2006;**49**:397-400

[15] Hussain A, Mhmood H, Nicholls J, El-Hasani S. Prevention of intra-abdominal abscess following laparoscopic appendectomy for perforated appendicitis: A prospective study. International Journal of Surgery. 2008;**6**:374-377

[16] Petrowsky H, Demartines N, Rousson V, Clavien PA. Evidence -based value of prophylactic drainage in gastrointestinal surgery. A systematic review and meta-analyses. Annals of Surgery. 2004;**240**:1074-1085

Diastasis Recti and Other Midline Defects: Totally Subcutaneous Endoscopic Approach

Pablo José Medina, Guido Luis Busnelli and
Walter Sebastián Nardi

Additional information is available at the end of the chapter

http://dx.doi.org/10.5772/intechopen.75653

Abstract

Diastasis of the rectus is defined as the separation of the midline or alba line, which originates in a laxity of the interlocking fibers from the aponeurosis of both rectus muscles. At present, its surgical correction continues to be discussed. However, there is a multiplicity of factors that justify it.

Keywords: diastasis recti, endoscopic rectus plication, mini-invasive, midline defects

1. Introduction

Diastasis recti is an anatomic term used to describe a condition in which both rectus muscles are separated by a distance greater than expected. Usually caused by the reduction of the consistency of the intercrossed fibers that make the linea alba, generating a separation of both aponeurosis of the rectus abdominis muscles. It can be congenital or acquired, favored by situations like pregnancy, obesity or previous surgeries.

Clinically represents an aesthetic and symptomatic problem. It produces malfunction of the abdominal wall muscles with an associated muscular imbalance and chronic back pain [1, 2].

Nowadays, there is no consensus on the surgical technique or indications for the treatment of diastasis recti, specially in patients without lipodystrophy. If is symptomatic, causes esthetic problems (specially in young women after pregnancy [3]) or associated with midline hernias (**Figure 1a–c**), the surgical treatment of both pathologies at the same time could be recommended. The most common technique used is by the way of an abdominoplasty

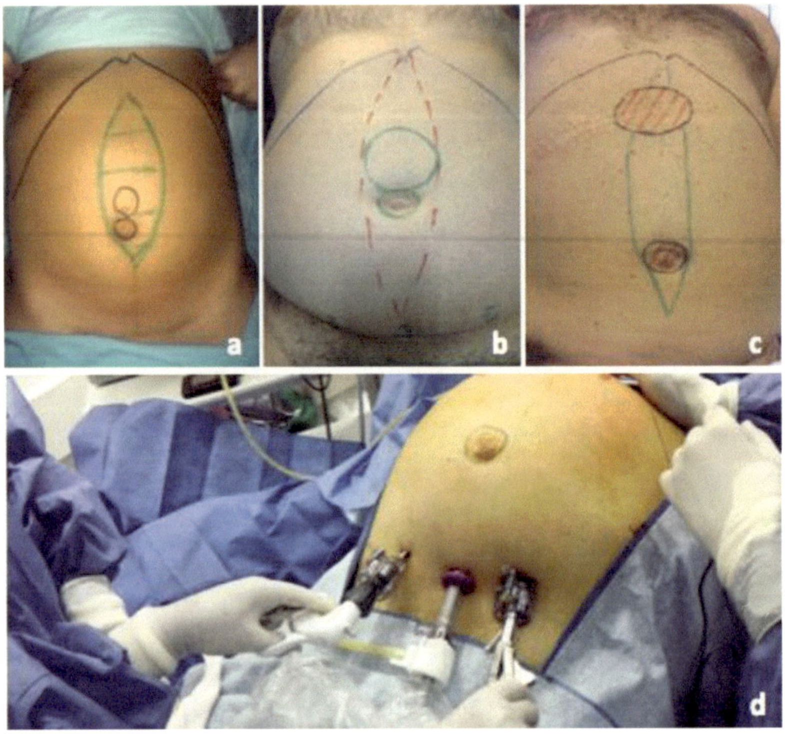

Figure 1. (a–c) External marking of the diastase recti and it's associated midline defects. (d) Position of the trocars and surgeon.

in patients with excess abdominal skin and subcutaneous cellular tissue [4]. However, a mini-invasive approach presents as an alternative procedure to the most commonly used technique for its treatment.

2. Surgical technique/technical aspects

Different options have been proposed such as conventional surgery, with abdominoplasty, laparoscopic or endoscopic approach.

For the endoscopic approach, under general anesthesia, the patient is positioned in supine position with both legs open and the surgeon is located between them. The monitor is located at the head of the patient and the assistant on his left. A 10 mm incision is made in the suprapubic midline and a space is created between the subcutaneous cellular tissue and the superficial aponeurosis with blunt dissection. A 10 mm trocar is introduced for the optic and, favored by a 10 mm Hg pneumatic pressure, two 5-mm trocars are placed under direct vision on each side of the midline by around 5 cm (**Figure 1d**).

10 mm Hg CO_2 is used to maintain a correct work space. Under endoscopic vision, the supra-aponeurotic space is dissected exposing the linea alba and superficial aponeurosis until

http://dx.doi.org/10.5772/intechopen.75653

reaching the umbilical region. The umbilicus is disinserted above the hernia sac if present, reintroducing it into the intra-abdominal compartment. If other supraumbilical abdominal wall defects are present, the dissection is done as previously described. Finally, the dissection of the supra-aponeurotic space continues until reaching the subxiphoid region. Once dissection is completed, the diastasis recti and associated aponeurotic defects can be identified (**Figure 2a** and **b**).

The plication of the aponeurosis of the recti muscles is done with two continuous absorbable barbed sutures from the subxiphoid to suprapubic region (**Figure 2c** and **d**).

In patients with associated large abdominal wall defects, the plication of both muscles can be difficult and the release of one or both rectus abdominis muscle aponeurosis could be convenient for a tension-free plication. The *component separation technique* allows a better compliance and 4–5 cm (each side) for the approximation of the muscles to the midline.

If the defect/s measures more than 4 cm, a prosthetic material is preferred to complete the abdominal wall repair. Usually, a polypropylene mesh is introduced in the supra-aponeurotic space (onlay) and fixed with knots of an absorbable suture or tracks (**Figure 3a–c**).

Finally, the umbilicus is reinserted to its normal position to the plicated fascia with an intracorporeal knotting (**Figure 3d**). Drainage is placed through one of the 5 mm wounds used in the surgery and a compressive bandage is used to decrease the dead space between the aponeurosis and the subcutaneous cellular tissue.

For the laparoscopic approach, the patient is placed supine with both arms outstretched. The monitor is located on the right flank. Pneumoperitoneum to 12 mm Hg is achieved via open

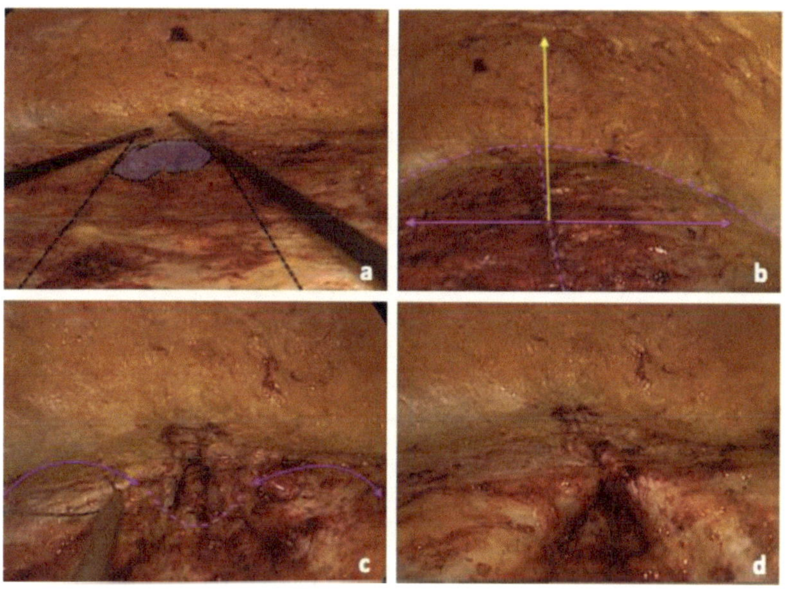

Figure 2. (a) Visualization of the diastasis recti and associated midline defect. (b) Final dissection of the supra-aponeurotic space until the subxifoid region. (c and d) Plication of the aponeurosis of diastase recti with absorbable barbed suture.

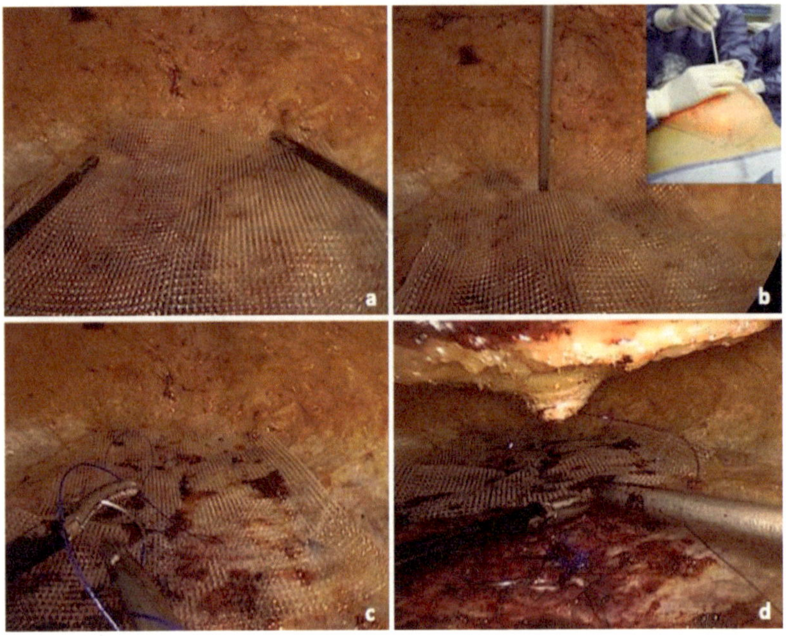

Figure 3. (a) Supra-aponeurotic polypropylene mesh is necessary to complete the abdominal wall repair. (b and c) Fixation with tracks and absorbable suture. (d) Reinsertion of the umbilicus with an intracorporeal knotting.

access of 12 mm in left flank and two additional trocars are placed in left upper quadrant (12 mm) and the left iliac fossa (5 mm).

Is better to start with laparoscopic time because sometimes is necessary to make extensive enterolysis and this is usually the most laborious process (**Figure 4**). All previous wall adhesions must be released.

Diastasis of rectus abdominis is observed and measured in all its extension (**Figure 5**).

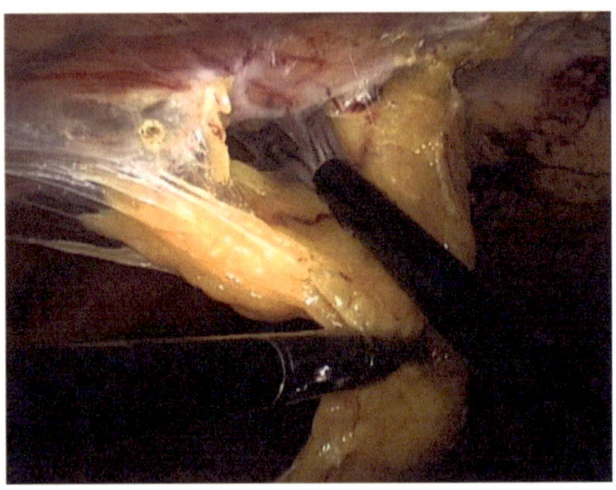

Figure 4. Release of anterior wall adhesions.

http://dx.doi.org/10.5772/intechopen.75653

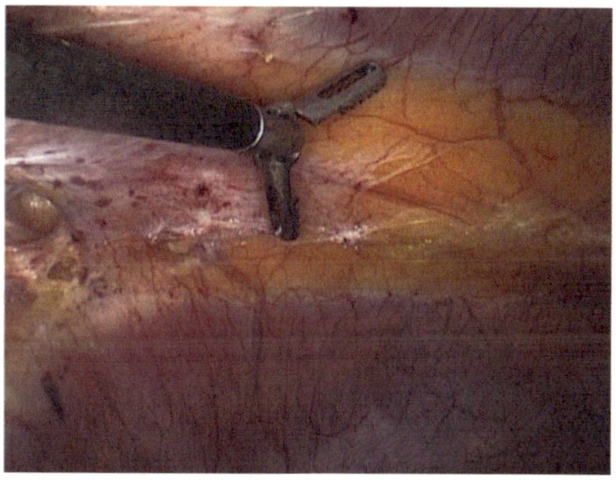

Figure 5. Measurement of diastasis recti using the diameter of the grasper.

Later on, some cases can use the *videoscopic component separation technique* to release rectus abdominis muscle and allow a tension-free plication. Exsufflation is performed and the same port sites are used. The external oblique muscle aponeurosis is identified in the upper 12 mm incision and is sectioned to access the avascular space between the external oblique and internal oblique muscles. This plane is developed with a blunt instrument. The space is then insufflated under vision and the semilunar line is visualized. The insufflation pressure is maintained at 12 mm Hg and the other two abdominal trocars are removed up to the space between both oblique muscles. This space is developed with blunt grasper maneuvers all the way between the costal margin and the inguinal ligament inferiorly. Finally, the release of the rectus is obtained by making an incision in the external oblique fascia lateral to the semilunar line. Hence, a release of the abdominis rectus sheath of about 6–8 cm is reached (**Figure 6a** and **b**). Is important to remember that nerve supply to the rectus muscle is medial to the semilunar line, hence the procedure prevents any injury to the nerves. If the diastasis is very large, greater than about 6 or 7 cm, the same procedure can be reproduced on the other side. Hemostasis is ensured and no drains are left in the dissected space. The abdominal cavity is then entered again.

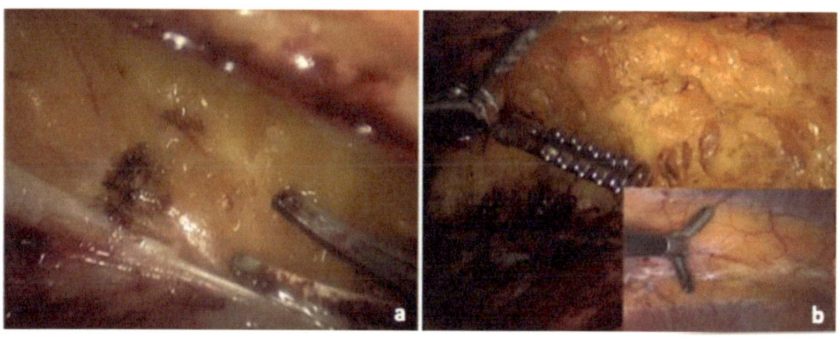

Figure 6. (a) Section of the external oblique aponeurosis. (b) Comparison between the distance between the external oblique fascia sectioned and the diameter of the diastasis.

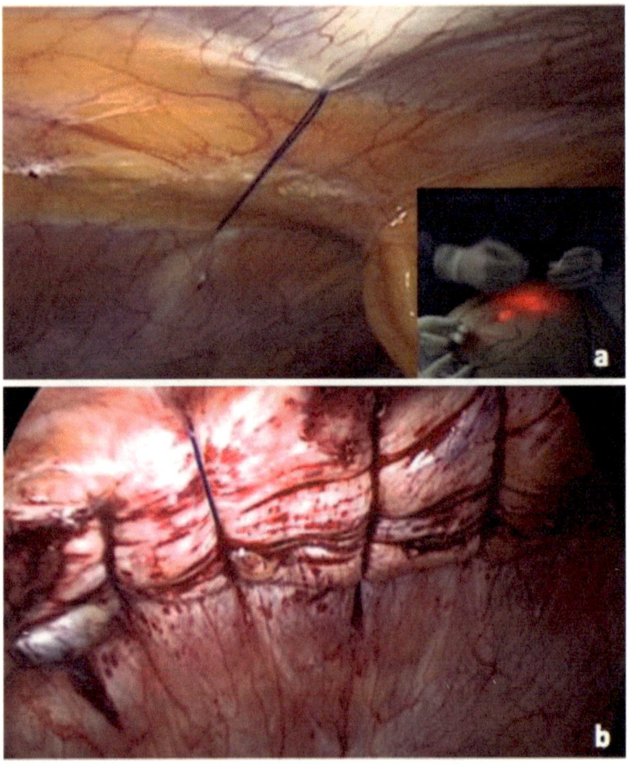

Figure 7. (a) and (b) Transmural stitches of polypropylene are placed along the entire diastasis including both rectus abdominis muscles with a laparoscopic suture passer device.

Transmural stitches of polypropylene suture are placed along the entire diastasis including both rectus abdominis muscles with a laparoscopic suture passer device such as "Endo Close™" (**Figure 7a** and **b**). Each stitch is introduced through a punctate stab incision in the skin and the knots are hidden in the subcutaneous tissue. After that, a composite mesh is prepared with permanent sutures that are placed at the midpoint of each side of the mesh before it is introduced into the abdominal cavity through a 12-mm trocar. Once the mesh is placed inside the abdominal cavity, it is secured to the abdominal wall with the preplaced sutures. Metal or absorbable tacks are then used circumferentially at approximately 1-cm intervals to prevent intestinal herniation.

3. Discussion

For the study of diastasis recti, CT scan or ultrasonography can be used. Both methods are reliable for the measurement of the separation of the rectus muscles. CT scan has the advantage of using bony ridges for that measurement and also can show other associated hernias [5]. Some authors propose that ultrasonography is an accurate method to measure rectus diastasis above the umbilicus and at the umbilical level. However, below umbilicus ultrasound can show smaller values [6].

Several ways to define and assess rectus muscle diastasis can be found in the literature. In addition, there is no consensus on the values considered relevant. Some authors consider any separation of the rectus abdominis as a diastasis and others consider a distance greater than 1 cm, 2 fingers or 3 cm.

The standard treatment of this condition is abdominoplasty with periumbilical incision, which often results in an umbilical circumcision or even an inverted T scar [7]. Limited incision abdominoplasty, sometimes called extended miniabdominoplasty, has been described in the literature but has received little attention. In conclusion, the majority of these techniques are for an open approach, while laparoscopy or endoscopy was not frequently reported at first. Nowadays plication of the diastasis without skin resection using only laparoscopic or endoscopic approach has been reported.

It is frequent to observe the coexistence of diastasis recti with one or more hernia or symptomatic incisional midline hernia. If only the hernia were treated, it would be done over an anatomic weak and deficient tissue, which is the damaged linea alba. This situation could lead to a higher possibility of hernia recurrence and also the aesthetic results would be uncertain. Thus, in these cases, simultaneous correction of all existent pathologies is highly recommended [8].

One option described for the plication of diastasis recti with skin resection is the laparoscopic approach [9]. Transmural stitches or even intracorporeal continuous suture can be done to reduce the diastasis. Finally an intra-peritoneal mesh is used to complete the procedure.

Bellido Luque et al. described the subcutaneous endoscopic approach as a new alternative to treat diastasis recti [4]. As explained before, with three supra-pubic trocars and using a pressure of CO_2 maintained between 8 and 10 mm Hg, a totally endoscopic treatment is used for the plicature of diastasis recti and also to treat associated abdominal wall defects. The utilization of barbed sutures for the plicature allows more rapid surgical maneuvers and therefore diminishing surgical times. Even though this suture is absorbable (180 days), a second continuous non-absorbable monofilament suture is added to ensure more stability [10].

Moreover, in some cases diastasis recti plicature, even though is effective, can lead to and excessive tension and therefore increased postoperative pain. In these cases, in our opinion, is necessary to reduce the rectus abdominis suture tension by dividing the external oblique muscle fascia close to the semilunar line and hence medializing the rectus abdominis muscle (*component separation*).

In 1990, Ramirez et al. described the "component separation" technique for the reconstruction of ventral hernias without the use of prosthetic material. Using this technique, up to 10 cm of unilateral recti advancement can be achieved.

On the other hand, it is well known that when an extensive dissection is needed to reach a "component separation", several complications are described (such as hematomas, wound infections, seromas, skin flaps necrosis, etc.). However, many studies report that an optimal compliance of the abdominal wall can be obtained by minimally invasive component separation. It provides up to 86% myofascial advancement compared with an open release [11]. Giurgius et al. compared the conventional component separation technique versus the mini invasive approach for ventral hernias. They concluded that the last one has advantages over the open technique due to a reduction in wound complications. The reduced incidence of seromas seen in the mini invasive approach is likely attributable to the ability to perform the procedure without the creation of undermining skin flaps.

The videoscopic component separation preserves the rectus abdominis myocutaneous perforators supplying the overlying skin and the connection between the subcutaneous fat and anterior rectus sheath, thereby reducing subcutaneous dead space and potentially improving overlying skin flap vascularity. In our opinion, this technique is not only useful for ventral hernia repairs, but also for abdominis diastasis recti surgery. The use of a reinforcing mesh aims to reduce the rate of recurrence.

4. Our experience and conclusion

A total of 42 patients underwent endoscopic surgery between March/2014 and Feb/2017 at British Hospital of Buenos Aires. Most of the patients (76%) were women with a mean age of 39 years and all of them (32) had a history of pregnancy. In 93% (39) of the cases, the diastasis was supra and infraumbilical and its average size was 5.5 cm (range 4–7 cm). About 100% of the patients had at least one associated abdominal wall defect, with the following distributions: 23 umbilical hernias, 18 epigastric hernias, 9 umbilical incisional hernias, and 1 subcostal incisional hernia. We had no intraoperative complications. The mean surgical time was 80 min (55–105 min). Polypropylene meshes were used in 38 patients (91%). Pain intensity at 12 h and at 7 postoperative days was evaluated by analogous visual scale (VAS) and was 4.1 points on average (range 1–6 pts.). The average degree of satisfaction with the cosmetic result was 9.5 with a range of 8–10. All the patients reported being very satisfied with the aesthetic and functional result and the procedure met their preoperative expectations.

Between the 8–10° postoperatory months, the abdominal wall was assessed by ultrasound in 39 patients (93%). After a follow-up of 7–35 months (mean, 10 months), we had no recurrences.

In conclusion, in patients without excess skin or subcutaneous cellular tissue, endoscopic approach to diastasis recti associated with midline hernias is a feasible and reproducible method. It has esthetic advantages, allowing simultaneous correction of all existent pathologies, with minimal complications. Diastasis recti measuring more than 6 cm may benefit with an additional videoscopic component separation technique and/or by using prosthetic mesh.

Laparoscopic approach is also another option for its repair. In this mini-invasive technique, using videoscopic component separation to decrease the tension of the suture between both rectus abdominis is the key to a proper reconstruction.

Author details

Pablo José Medina, Guido Luis Busnelli and Walter Sebastián Nardi*

*Address all correspondence to: nardi.ws@gmail.com

British Hospital of Buenos Aires, Buenos Aires, Argentina

References

[1] Carreirao S, Correa WE, Dias LC, Pitanguy I. Treatment of abdominal wall eventrations associated with abdominoplasty techniques. Aesthetic Plastic Surgery. 1984;**8**(3):173-179

[2] Ramirez OM. Abdominoplasty and abdominal wall rehabilitation: Comprehensive approach. Plastic and Reconstructive Surgery. 2000;**105**(1):425-435

[3] Beer GM, Schuster A, Seifert B, Manestar M, Mihic-Probst DA, Weber SA. The normal width of the linea alba in nulliparous women. Clinical Anatomy. 2009;**22**:706-711

[4] Bellido Luque J, Bellido Luque A, Valdivia J, Suarez Gráu JM, Gomez Menchero J, et al. Totally endoscopic surgery on diastasis recti associated with midline hernias. The advantages of a minimally invasive approach. Prospective cohort study. Hernia. 2015;**19**(3):493-501

[5] Nahas FX, Ferreira LM, Augusto SM. Ghelfond. Long-term follow-up of correction of rectus diastasis. Plastic and Reconstructive Surgery. 2015;**115**(6):1736-1741

[6] Mendes Dde A, Nahas FX, Veiga DF. Ultrasonography for measuring rectus abdominis muscles diastasis. Acta Cirúrgica Brasileira. 2007;**22**:182-186

[7] Yousif NJ, Lifchez SD, Nguyen HH. Transverse rectus sheath plication in abdominoplasty. Plastic and Reconstructive Surgery. 2004;**114**:778

[8] Al-Qattan M. Abdominoplasty in multiparous women with severe musculoaponeurotic laxity. British Journal of Plastic Surgery. 1997;**50**:450-455

[9] Champault G. Video-laparoscopic surgery of the abdominal wall. A study of 15 cases. Chirurgie. 2004;**123**(5):474-477

[10] Rosen A. Repair of the midline fascial defect in abdominoplasty with long-acting barbed and smooth absorbable sutures. Aesthetic Surgery Journal. 2011;**31**(6):668-673

[11] Rosen MJ, Williams C, Jin J, McGee MF, Schomisch S, Marks J, Ponsky J. Laparoscopic versus open-component separation: A comparative analysis in porcine model. American Journal of Surgery. 2007;**194**(3):385-389

Chapter 3

Robotic Hysterectomy for Cancer and Benign Pathology

Adrian Kohut, Leah Goldberg and
Alexandre Buckley De Meritens

Additional information is available at the end of the chapter

http://dx.doi.org/10.5772/intechopen.76466

Abstract

The da Vinci Surgical System is an innovative technology that has advanced the laparoscopic treatment of benign and malignant diseases in gynecology. In this chapter, we will discuss the da Vinci Surgical System technology, including its history, utilization, surgical technique for benign and oncologic hysterectomy, future directions and surgical complications. Through a review of the literature, we aim to chronicle the current trends of application in both benign and oncologic gynecologic conditions and describe the current standards of care in this innovative and evolving operative technology. Although the future utility of robotic surgeries and robotic hysterectomies necessitates further research, the potential application of this surgical method affords great promise.

Keywords: robotic hysterectomy, gynecologic oncology, benign gynecologic surgery

1. History

The initial da Vinci robotic surgical system (Intuitive Surgical, Sunnyvale, CA) was released in Europe in 1999 and received FDA approval in 2000 [1]. In 2005, the FDA approved the da Vinci robotic system for gynecological surgeries. The first system consisted of two robotic operating arms and one camera holder. Since its emergence in the surgical arena, there have been four updates to the system, each of which has increased its overall capability within various surgical subspecialties and overall maneuverability of instrument use. The latest version termed the da Vinci Xi was released in 2014 and includes 3D HD vision, four quadrant mounting, and instruments capable of moving in seven degrees of motion while performing complex surgical techniques including clamping, cutting, coagulating, dissecting, suturing and manipulating tissue [2].

In 2002, Diaz-Arrastia et al. published a series of 11 patients undergoing uncomplicated da Vinci assisted total laparoscopic hysterectomy and bilateral salpingo-oophorectomy demonstrating feasibility for its use in gynecologic surgery [3]. Subsequently, Lambaudie et al. published a report of 28 patients undergoing various da Vinci assisted surgical procedures for gynecologic cancer including total hysterectomy, bilateral oophorectomy, and pelvic and/or para-aortic lymphadenectomy. The authors found that the use of robot-assisted laparoscopy led to less intraoperative blood loss, less postoperative pain and shorter hospital stays compared with those treated with more traditional surgical approaches such as laparoscopy and laparotomy [4]. The following year the FDA approved the use of the da Vinci robotic system for use in gynecologic oncology surgery.

2. Introduction

Over the past 12 years, the da Vinci assisted approach to laparoscopic hysterectomy has taken a more prominent role in the surgical management of a multitude of benign and oncologic gynecologic conditions. Multiple meta-analyses and literature reviews have shown that the use of robotic surgery offers the advantage of decreased blood loss and length of stay when compared to open surgical techniques [5]. When compared to traditional laparoscopic methods outcomes appear to be equivocal, but a case can be made for the advantages of robotic surgery to treat obese patients [6]. The main disadvantages of robotic gynecologic surgery include increased intraoperative time and cost-effectiveness questionability. Such issues may be mitigated as operator proficiency increases. Future projections of advancement in robotic gynecologic surgery highlight the use of minimal incisions and single site approaches [7].

Hysterectomy is one of the most frequently performed surgical procedures in the United States. Common benign indications include symptomatic uterine leiomyomas (51.4%), abnormal uterine bleeding (41.7%), endometriosis (30%), and prolapse (18.2%) [8, 9].

The American College of Obstetricians and Gynecologists favors vaginal hysterectomy as the preferred method among women undergoing hysterectomy for benign disease [10]. A 2015 Cochrane Database Systematic Review indicated that vaginal hysterectomy appears to be superior to both laparoscopic hysterectomy and abdominal hysterectomy as it is associated with faster return to normal activities [11]. However, in cases involving factors such as adnexal pathology, severe endometriosis, adhesions, or an enlarged uterus, vaginal hysterectomy may not be appropriate [10]. Compared to abdominal hysterectomy, laparoscopic hysterectomy is associated with decreased risk of perioperative complications, faster return to normal activity, decreased length of hospital stay, decreased risk of readmission, decreased risk of surgical site infection, decreased blood loss and need for blood transfusion, and improved postoperative quality of life [11]. Though current evidence demonstrates a less significant difference between robot-assisted laparoscopic hysterectomy and conventional laparoscopic hysterectomy, potential benefits of the robotic-assisted approach include decreased complication rate, decreased length of hospital stay, decreased blood loss and need for blood transfusion, and decreased risk of conversion to exploratory laparotomy for surgically complicated cases and obese patients [9, 12–19]. With an increasing number of both academic institutions and community hospitals offering robotic surgery, there is a national uptrend in rates of the robotic-assisted approach. Of all benign hysterectomies, robotic-assisted surgery increased from 0.5% in 2007 to 9.5% in 2010 [9, 13, 18, 20–27].

In the context of gynecologic oncology, common indications for hysterectomy include cancers of the endometrium, cervix, ovary or fallopian tube. The 2017 NCCN Clinical Practice Guidelines in Oncology for Uterine Neoplasm state that "Minimally invasive hysterectomy is now the preferred approach when technically feasible" [28]. The randomized controlled trial LAP2 showed short-term surgical benefits of laparoscopy over laparotomy for uterine cancer staging, and follow-up data showed equivalent oncologic outcomes [29]. In the case of cervical cancer, even though we do not have phase III data supporting the use of minimally invasive surgery, there is a body of literature demonstrating feasibility and suggesting equivalent oncologic outcomes compared to abdominal hysterectomy [30–32].

Robotic surgery has taken center stage in becoming the standard of care in patients with early-stage endometrial and cervical cancer. When comparing robotic-assisted surgery with conventional laparoscopy for endometrial cancer, robotic surgery has been found to have decreased length of stay, reduced operating time, decreased blood loss, and more rapid post-surgical recovery [6]. Furthermore, robotic surgery has even been shown to result in high lymph note count as compared to conventional laparoscopy when performed in obese women with endometrial cancer [33]. In comparing robot-assisted surgery with abdominal surgery for endometrial cancer, robotic surgery is associated with decreased blood loss, reduced length of stay, increased operation duration, and equal number of lymph node counts [20, 34–40]. In analyzing total cost of care for endometrial cancer patients, robotic surgery has been shown to be significantly cheaper ($8212.00 versus $12,943.60, P = .001) due to its association with a decreased length of stay [20, 34, 41]. In patients with early cervical cancer, robotic-assisted and conventional laparoscopic radical hysterectomy have both been shown to be superior to exploratory laparotomy due to decreased blood loss, decreased complication rates, reduced the length of stay, and increased lymph node count. In such patients, there is conflicting data showing the advantage of the robotic approach over conventional laparoscopy [36, 42–58]. There is currently limited data on the use of robotics in the setting of advanced ovarian cancer, and thus its use is not recommended at this time [3, 4, 59–63].

In this chapter, we will describe the technology behind the robotic-assisted surgery, patient preparation, surgical technique for simple and radical hysterectomy and complications.

3. The technology

Robot-assisted laparoscopy is an innovative advancement in gynecologic laparoscopic surgery. The robotic approach enhances traditional laparoscopy by providing three-dimensional optics, advanced ergonomics, improved vision and precision, tremor filtration, and 7° of motion with advanced dexterity [2]. There are currently four generations of the da Vinci Surgical System: The "standard", the S, the Si, the X and the Xi system. The components of the da Vinci Surgical System include the surgeon console, the patient side cart, and the vision system [2] (**Figure 1**).

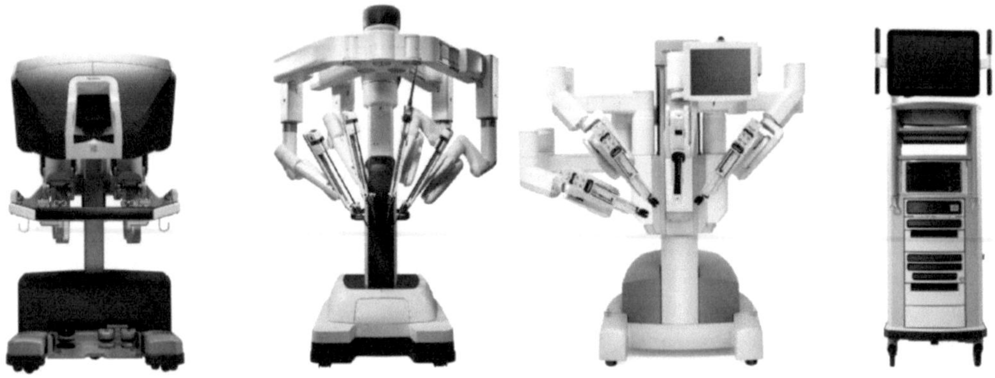

a b c

Figure 1. (a) Surgeons console; (b) patients side-cart; and (c) vision tower.

The surgeon operates seated at the console while viewing a 3D high-definition image inside the patient's body. The surgeon's fingers grasp the master controls below the display which converts the surgeon's hand, wrist and finger movements into precise, simultaneous movements of surgical instruments [2].

The patient-side cart is where the patient is positioned during surgery. Attached to the side cart are four robotic arms that facilitate the surgeon's commands by moving around fixed pivot points which allow for less force on the abdominal wall than laparoscopy [2]. The vision system is equipped with a 3D, high-definition endoscope and image processing equipment for visualization of the patient's anatomy [2]. A view of the operating field is available to the entire OR team on a large viewing monitor (vision cart) [2].

A full range of EndoWrist instruments (Intuitive Surgical, Sunnyvale, CA) is available to the surgeon while operating. Most instruments are modeled after the human wrist, offering a greater range of motion than the human hand. Each instrument is designed for a particular task, such as clamping, cutting, coagulating, dissecting, suturing and manipulating tissue. EndoWrist Instruments feature 7° of freedom, 90° of articulation, natural motion and fingertip control, motion scaling and tremor reduction [2]. Energy instruments include da Vinci monopolar and bipolar cautery instruments (electrical energy), the da Vinci Harmonic™ ACE (mechanical energy), the da Vinci PK™ Dissecting Forceps (advanced bipolar), and laser [2]. Grasping instruments allow handling thin, delicate tissues as well as thicker and stronger tissues. Needle drivers provide the ability to suture with fine and thick needles. SutureCut™ Needle Drivers include a cutting blade for efficient cutting of suture after knot tying [2].

4. Indications

Robotic hysterectomy may be employed for a wide spectrum of benign pathologies including leiomyoma, abnormal uterine bleeding, endometriosis, adenomyosis, adnexal mass, pelvic pain, and pelvic organ prolapse. Common malignant pathologies necessitating hysterectomy include primary cancers of the uterus, ovary, cervix, fallopian tubes, and peritoneum; as well as nongynecologic metastases of urologic, colorectal, breast, gastrointestinal, renal, pulmonary, melanomatous, or lymphatic origin.

5. Technique

After induction of general endotracheal anesthesia and insertion of an orogastric tube, the patient is placed in dorsal lithotomy position using yellowfin stirrups with careful padding of pressure points. Both arms are padded and tucked to the sides. The patient is placed in steep Trendelenburg position (27–30°) to allow mobilization of the small bowel out the pelvic area and exposing the aorta if in need to perform lymph node dissection. She is prepped and draped in the standard sterile fashion. Foley catheter is inserted, and a uterine manipulator such as a V-care manipulator (ConMed Endosurgery, Utica, NY) or the Advincula Arch uterine manipulator (Cooper Surgical, Trumbull, CT) is placed. The uterine manipulator allows demarcation of the cervicovaginal junction necessary to perform the colpotomy.

5.1. Port placement

Port placement can differ based on uterine size, the need to do lymph node dissection, using 2 or 3 operative arms and the da Vinci system used (**Figure 2**). The endoscope port is the reference port for all other ports. If not doing lymph node dissection and with a small uterus, the camera port can be placed 8–10 cm above the fundus which ends up being at the umbilicus. For oncologic surgery, we place the camera port 20–25 cm above the pubic bone [64]. When using the S or Si system we place a 10–12 mm laparoscopic port for the camera and when using the Xi system we place the 8 mm da Vinci camera trocar. The ports need to be 6–10 cm apart to allow triangulation and avoid arms collision. When using three operative arms, the surgeon can decide to place the third arm either at the right or left hemi-abdomen. Placing the third operative arm on the right will result in controlling both arms with the surgeon's right hand and vice versa if placed on the left hemi-abdomen.

When using the Xi system the operative ports can be placed in a straight line at the level of the umbilicus but all ports can be shifted up for a large uterus or for lymph node dissection. The assist port is usually placed 2–3 cm under the left rib cage over the mid-clavicular line (Palmer point) but can be place in the lower quadrants. Careful placement should be done to avoid placing the assistant port in a straight line with the target anatomy and an operative port. This would result in difficult access to the surgical field for the assistant. We like using either a 5 or 8 mm Airseal trocar for the assist port (ConMed Utica, NY). When using the S or Si systems operative ports should be placed 8–10 cm apart and keeping 10–20 cm distance to the target anatomy.

5.2. Docking the patient-side cart

For gynecologic surgery, docking can be done either between the patient's legs or from the side (**Figure 3**). We like side docking because it allows for an assistant to occupy the space between

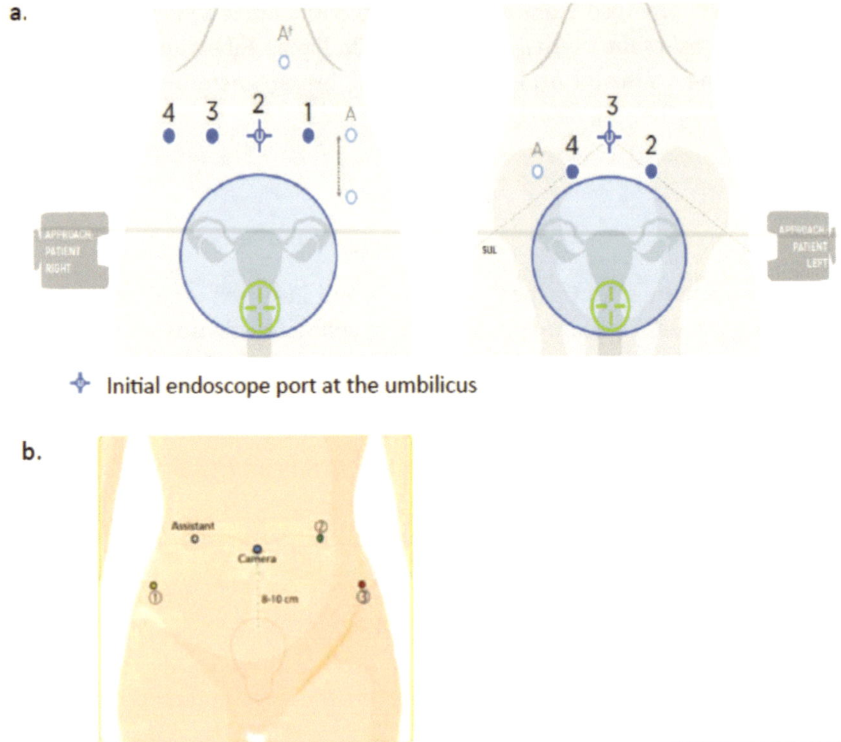

Figure 2. (a) Port placement for the Xi system showing 3 operative arms and 2 operative arms configuration and (b) port placement for the S and Si systems.

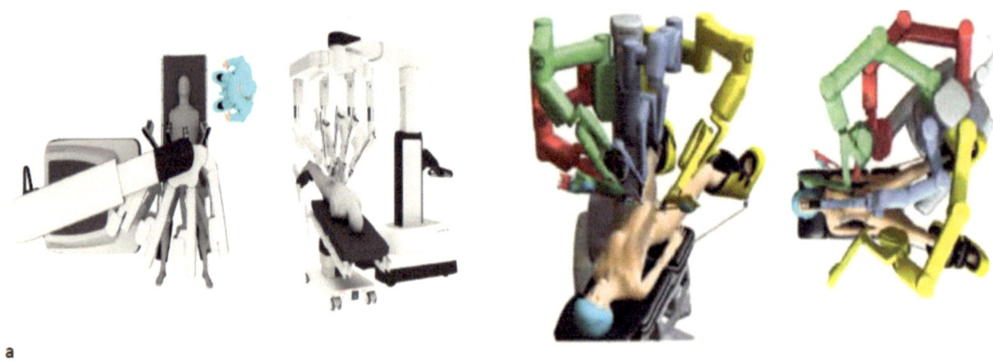

Figure 3. Side docking. Side docking with the Xi and S system.

the legs and use the uterine manipulator and deliver specimens through the vagina without difficulty. When using the S system, the robotic column is positioned at a 45° acute angle relative to the cephalad/caudal axis of the patient. When using the Xi system the patient-side cart can be approached in almost any angle to the bed and the arms are rotated to fix their position.

5.3. Simple hysterectomy technique

A survey of the entire abdominal cavity is performed laparoscopically. Once the robotic column is successfully docked bipolar forceps are inserted into the left-sided instrument port, monopolar scissors are inserted into the right-sided instrument port, and a grasper inserted into the rightmost port. The assistant seated at the left upper quadrant assistant port starts the procedure with a suction irrigator, laparoscopic bowel grasper, laparoscopic Maryland, and laparoscopic scissors all on hand.

The pelvic peritoneum is incised parallel to the infundibulopelvic ligament. The external iliac artery is identified and traced down to the bifurcation of the common iliac artery. The ureter is found entering the pelvis at the level of the bifurcation. At this point, the ovarian vessels contained in the infundibulopelvic ligament are isolated from the ureter by creating a window in the posterior sheet of the broad ligament. Either the ovarian vessels are clamped, cauterized and transected if a salpingo-oophorectomy is intended or the utero-ovarian ligament. The posterior sheet of the broad ligament is extended in the direction of the uterosacral ligament skeletonizing the uterine artery. The round ligament is then clamped, cauterized and transected. The anterior sheet of the broad ligament is opened in the direction of the vesicouterine peritoneal reflexion. After performing this procedure bilaterally, the bladder is mobilized off of the upper vagina to expose the cervicovaginal junction marked by the colpotomizer of the uterine manipulator. The uterine vessels are then clamped, cauterized and transected at a 90° angle at the cervico-uterine junction. The cardinal ligament is then clamped, cauterized and transected medially to the uterine vessel pedicle and parallel to the cervix. After performing the colpotomy, the specimen is delivered through the vagina. A sterile glove filled with a lap sponge is inserted into the vagina once the specimen is successfully extracted to maintain adequate pneumoperitoneum. The vaginal cuff is then closed using either one polysorb or v-lock suture.

5.4. Radical hysterectomy

The surgical technique is similar to the traditional Type III abdominal radical hysterectomy. The avascular spaces (pararectal, paravesical and obturator spaces) are developed to identify the ureters, the major vessels (external and interior iliac arteries, the superior vesical and uterine arteries), the obturator nerve and the genitofemoral nerve (**Figure 4**). The uterine artery is cauterized and transected at its origin and mobilized medially to expose the ureter. Complete ureterolysis is performed to the canal of Wertheim, and the ureter is then unroofed allowing to mobilize both the ureter and the bladder away from the upper third of the vagina. The peritoneum between both uterosacral ligaments is incised, and the paravesical space is bluntly developed, thus allowing transection of the uterosacral ligament at its origin. The paracolpos is then clamped, cauterized and transected parallel to the vagina allowing to perform the upper vaginectomy.

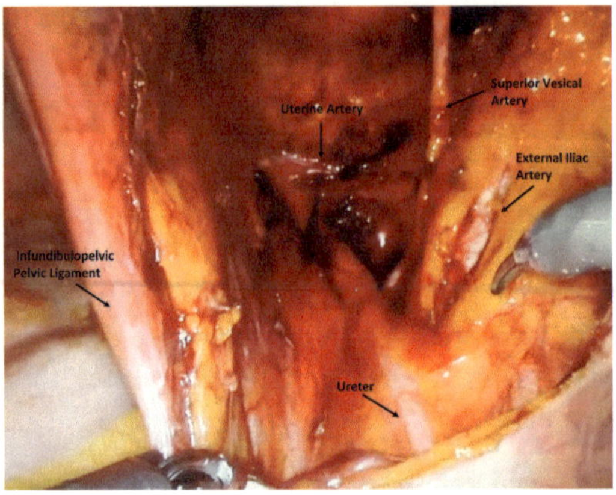

Figure 4. Right retroperitoneal pelvic sidewall anatomy.

6. Future robotic surgery

6.1. Multiport and single port

Single port laparoscopy is a relatively new advancement in minimally invasive surgery. Da Vinci surgery with Single-Site has been approved for cholecystectomy, hysterectomy, and salpingo-oophorectomy in benign conditions. Traditional or robotic-assisted single port laparoscopy for hysterectomy and other gynecologic procedures such as myomectomy and adnexal surgery has been reported in the literature with favorable outcomes [65–67]. Known advantages include improved cosmetic appearance as there is only one incision, decrease postoperative pain and wound infection, and minimization of potential damage to vasculature during port placement [68, 69]. However, single port laparoscopy has technical difficulties including instrument crowding leading to increased collision between instruments and limited degree of movement. There is also an increased risk of an incision-site hernia with single-port surgery. The da Vinci with Single-site technology for a hysterectomy requires a multichannel access port with an insufflation valve and space for four cannulas. Two curved ports are for the robotic controlled instruments, one port holds the endoscope, and the final one is the designated assistant port. In the current literature, there are only retrospective study designs that compare single port laparoscopy with multiport while using the da Vinci robotic system. Paek et al. compared surgical outcomes of single robotic site (n = 25) and laparoendoscopic single-site total hysterectomy (n = 442) for benign disease states [70]. The study found that the robotic group had a lower complication rate, and less operative bleeding, however, there was significantly longer operating times when compared to the laparoscopic group. Lopez et al. also found an increase in total operative time (approximately 25 min) while using the robotic-assisted single site compared to laparoscopic single site [71]. In this study, there was a significant decrease in length of hospital stay by 8 h in the robotic arm. Gungor et al. compared the operative time, perioperative and early operative complication rate, conversion to another technique rate, postoperative pain, and recovery time, and found that there were no significant differences between single site laparoscopy vs. robotic hysterectomy for benign disease [72]. Single site robotic and laparoscopic surgery was deemed to be safe and feasible techniques for total hysterectomy. In the hands of an experienced robotic surgeon, the learning curve of robotic laparoendoscopic single site surgery is fast, requiring 13 cases significantly decrease operative time [73]. While single port robotic-assisted hysterectomy seems promising, a Cochrane review reports that there is a lack of evidence of any benefit of a single port or robot-assisted hysterectomy when compared to traditional multi-port laparoscopic hysterectomy [11]. Future randomized control trials are needed to evaluate the potential advantages of robotic single site surgery.

7. Surgical complications

New causes of complication have been introduced with robotic-assisted surgery, but the overall incidence of complications is similar to those of conventional laparoscopic surgery. The FDA database reports 21% of injuries attributed to operator-related error and 14% to technical system failure [74]. The main drawback from robotic-assisted surgery is the loss of tactile feedback that can result in complications from poor tissue handling, blunt dissection of dense adhesions or inappropriate tying of sutures [75]. Other causes of complications in robotic-assisted surgery are note keeping the instruments in view, defects in protective sheaths of the shears, collision of instruments, poor positioning of the patient, port and trocar placement, vaginal vault dehiscence and cuff infection, and lack of communication within the team.

Steep Trendelenburg is often required to expose the pelvic anatomy and the para-aortic area during oncologic surgery. Prolonged Trendelenburg can result in mild head contusion, subcutaneous ecchymosis, orbital pain and peri-orbital edema, corneal abrasion, visual loss, laryngeal edema, nerve injuries. Reducing operative time or reversing Trendelenburg after 4–5 h, restrictive fluid replacement, adequate padding at pressure points can prevent some of these complications [75].

Specific organ injuries during robotic-assisted surgery have a similar incidence than during laparoscopic surgery. A systematic review of the literature comparing robotic surgery to laparotomy and conventional laparoscopy for cervical cancer shows comparable risk of urologic injuries (less than 1% bladder injuries and less than 3% ureteric injuries) [76]. Urologic injuries can be prevented by thoroughly identifying the ureter and careful surgical technique avoiding excessive devascularization of the ureter and excessive use of the cautery. The use of prophylactic stents in conventional laparoscopy and laparotomy has not shown to be cost effective for the prevention of urologic injury and has not been studied in robotic-assisted gynecologic surgery [77, 78]. Bowel and vascular injuries have a low incidence and similar causes than conventional laparoscopic surgery. Some preventive measures can be used to reduce injury during entrance to the abdominal cavity but no specific technique (veress needle, open technique) has shown to be superior to prevent injuries. Good surgical technique with good exposure and correct use of electric energy are important to prevent injuries. The majority of bowel injuries are recognized intra-operatively (87%) and repaired by minimally invasive approach (58%) [79]. Nerve injuries can occur due to poor patient positioning but also during lymph node dissection (genitofemoral nerve, obturator nerve) and parametrial dissection (para-sympathetic plexus) during radical hysterectomy. Although vaginal cuff dehiscence is uncommon, it is more prevalent in robotic surgery than conventional laparoscopy, laparotomy and vaginal surgery. It is reported in up to 1.5% of hysterectomies done for benign disease and up to 2.5% for oncologic disease [80, 81]. Several measures are recommended to limit the incidence of vaginal cuff dehiscence like the use of cutting mode electrocautery during the colpotomy to reduce thermal injury, incorporating 5 mm of healthy tissue from the vaginal edge, incorporating the posterior peritoneum and uterosacral ligaments for better support and avoiding vaginal trauma (intercourse, tampons, Valsalva) for 6–12 weeks [75]. In a review of the United States Food and Drug Administration (FDA) Manufacture and User Device Experience (MAUDE) Database reporting of gynecologic robotic procedures (the majority of which consisted of robotic hysterectomy) for the year 2012, risk of major operative injury was 0.08% and the risk of death was 0.007% [82].

8. Information for patients

Patients should be provided instructions regarding perioperative information and expectations. Patients should remain NPO starting at the 12 am hour before surgery. Bowel preparation is not necessary unless bowel resection is anticipated. Prior to proceeding to the operating room patients will review and sign procedure consents with their surgeon. Detailed information regarding possible intraoperative complications is detailed above in Section 7. In general patients should be made aware that risks of robotic assisted laparoscopic hysterectomy include but not be limited to vascular injury, hemorrhage, infection, injury to bowel, bladder, ureters, nerves, and other structures adjacent to the operative field. Patients should be informed that the risk of major morbidity and death are both small (approximately <1% and <0.01% respectively) [82]. In some cases reoperation with additional surgical interventions such as bowel resection with reanastamosis and/or diversion and ureteral reimplantation may be necessary. Major causes of postoperative morbidity include sepsis and venous thromboembolism. Prophylactic antibiotics and pharmacologic anticoagulation are often administered to minimize these risks. The majority of patients undergoing robotic hysterectomy are discharged home within 24–48 h of surgery, with a large portion of patients going home on the same day as surgery.

9. Conclusion

The da Vinci Surgical System is an innovative technology that has advanced the laparoscopic treatment of benign and malignant diseases in gynecology. Da Vinci assisted laparoscopic hysterectomy has advantages over open, traditional laparoscopic, and even vaginal approaches in some cases. This surgical technique is proliferating and being adopted by university and community hospitals across the country. As the literature on the benefits of da Vinci assisted hysterectomy continues to grow, so does operator proficiency and its use in operating rooms. The newer da Vinci models have increased movement efficiency and visual capacity. Although the future utility of robotic surgeries and robotic hysterectomies necessitates further research, the potential application of this surgical method affords great promise.

Author details

Adrian Kohut[1], Leah Goldberg[1] and Alexandre Buckley De Meritens[1,2]*

*Address all correspondence to: ab1641@cinj.rutgers.edu

1 Department of Obstetrics, Gynecology, and Reproductive Sciences, Rutgers Robert Wood Johnson Medical School, Robert Wood Johnson University Hospital, New Brunswick, NJ, United States

2 Division of Gynecologic Oncology, Rutgers Cancer Institute of New Jersey, Robert Wood Johnson University Hospital, New Brunswick, NJ, United States

References

[1] Ballantyne GH, Moll F. The da Vinci telerobotic surgical system: The virtual operative field and telepresence surgery. The Surgical Clinics of North America. 2003;**83**(6):1293-1304 vii

[2] Intuitive Surgical, I. The da Vinci Surgical System. 2017. Available from: https://intuitivesurgical.com/products/davinci_surgical_system/ [cited 2017]

[3] Diaz-Arrastia C et al. Laparoscopic hysterectomy using a computer-enhanced surgical robot. Surgical Endoscopy. 2002;**16**(9):1271-1273

[4] Lambaudie E et al. Robot-assisted laparoscopy in gynecologic oncology. Surgical Endoscopy. 2008;**22**(12):2743-2747

[5] Lauterbach R, Matanes E, Lowenstein L. Review of robotic surgery in gynecology—The future is here. Rambam Maimonides Medical Journal. 2017;**8**(2):1-12

[6] Gala RB et al. Systematic review of robotic surgery in gynecology: Robotic techniques compared with laparoscopy and laparotomy. Journal of Minimally Invasive Gynecology. 2014;**21**(3):353-361

[7] Moukarzel LA, Fader AN, Tanner EJ. Feasibility of robotic-assisted laparoendoscopic single-site surgery in the gynecologic oncology setting. Journal of Minimally Invasive Gynecology. 2017;**24**(2):258-263

[8] Whiteman MK et al. Inpatient hysterectomy surveillance in the United States, 2000-2004. American Journal of Obstetrics and Gynecology. 2008;**198**(1):34e1-34e7

[9] Wright JD et al. Robotically assisted vs laparoscopic hysterectomy among women with benign gynecologic disease. JAMA. 2013;**309**(7):689-698

[10] Committee on Gynecologic, P. Committee Opinion No 701: Choosing the Route of Hysterectomy for Benign Disease. Obstetrics and Gynecology. 2017;**129**(6):e155-e159

[11] Aarts JW et al. Surgical approach to hysterectomy for benign gynaecological disease. Cochrane Database of Systematic Reviews. 2015;**8**:CD003677

[12] Ho C et al. In Robot-Assisted Surgery Compared with Open Surgery and Laparoscopic Surgery: Clinical Effectiveness and Economic Analyses. Ottawa, ON: Canadian Agency for Drugs and Technologies in Health. 2011

[13] Landeen LB et al. Clinical and cost comparisons for hysterectomy via abdominal, standard laparoscopic, vaginal and robot-assisted approaches. South Dakota Medicine. 2011;**64**(6):197-199, 201, 203 passim

[14] Geppert B, Lonnerfors C, Persson J. Robot-assisted laparoscopic hysterectomy in obese and morbidly obese women: Surgical technique and comparison with open surgery. Acta Obstetricia et Gynecologica Scandinavica. 2011;**90**(11):1210-1217

[15] Lim PC et al. Multicenter analysis comparing robotic, open, laparoscopic, and vaginal hysterectomies performed by high-volume surgeons for benign indications. International Journal of Gynaecology and Obstetrics. 2016;**133**(3):359-364

[16] Scandola M et al. Robot-assisted laparoscopic hysterectomy vs traditional laparoscopic hysterectomy: Five metaanalyses. Journal of Minimally Invasive Gynecology. 2011;**18**(6):705-715

[17] Orady M et al. Comparison of robotic-assisted hysterectomy to other minimally invasive approaches. JSLS. 2012;**16**(4):542-548

[18] Rosero EB et al. Comparison of robotic and laparoscopic hysterectomy for benign gynecologic disease. Obstetrics and Gynecology. 2013;**122**(4):778-786

[19] Surgical I. da Vinci Xi Surgical System. 2017. Available from: https://www.intuitivesurgical.com/products/da-vinci-xi/ [cited 9/29/2017]

[20] Committee opinion no. 628: Robotic surgery in gynecology. Obstetrics and Gynecology. 2015;**125**(3):760-7

[21] Sarlos D et al. Robotic hysterectomy versus conventional laparoscopic hysterectomy: Outcome and cost analyses of a matched case-control study. European Journal of Obstetrics, Gynecology, and Reproductive Biology. 2010;**150**(1):92-96

[22] Matthews CA et al. Evaluation of the introduction of robotic technology on route of hysterectomy and complications in the first year of use. American Journal of Obstetrics and Gynecology. 2010;**203**(5):499e1-499e5

[23] Payne TN, Dauterive FR. A comparison of total laparoscopic hysterectomy to robotically assisted hysterectomy: Surgical outcomes in a community practice. Journal of Minimally Invasive Gynecology. 2008;**15**(3):286-291

[24] Kilic GS et al. Comparison of perioperative outcomes of total laparoscopic and robotically assisted hysterectomy for benign pathology during introduction of a robotic program. Obstetrics and Gynecology International. 2011;**2011**:683703

[25] Shashoua AR, Gill D, Locher SR. Robotic-assisted total laparoscopic hysterectomy versus conventional total laparoscopic hysterectomy. JSLS. 2009;**13**(3):364-369

[26] Nezhat C et al. Laparoscopic hysterectomy with and without a robot: Stanford experience. JSLS. 2009;**13**(2):125-128

[27] Yamasato K et al. Effect of robotic surgery on hysterectomy trends: Implications for resident education. Journal of Minimally Invasive Gynecology. 2014;**21**(3):399-405

[28] Network NCC. NCCN Clinical Practice Guidelines in Oncology: Uterine Neoplasms. 2016

[29] Walker JL et al. Recurrence and survival after random assignment to laparoscopy versus laparotomy for comprehensive surgical staging of uterine cancer: Gynecologic Oncology Group LAP2 Study. Journal of Clinical Oncology. 2012;**30**(7):695-700

[30] Zhao Y et al. Laparoscopic radical hysterectomy in early stage cervical cancer: A systematic review and meta-analysis. Journal of Laparoendoscopic & Advanced Surgical Techniques. Part A. 2017;**27**(11):1132-1144

[31] Bogani G et al. Laparoscopic versus open abdominal management of cervical cancer: Long-term results from a propensity-matched analysis. Journal of Minimally Invasive Gynecology. 2014;**21**(5):857-862

[32] Liu Z et al. Superiority of robotic surgery for cervical cancer in comparison with traditional approaches: A systematic review and meta-analysis. International Journal of Surgery. 2017;**40**:145-154

[33] Gehrig PA et al. What is the optimal minimally invasive surgical procedure for endometrial cancer staging in the obese and morbidly obese woman? Gynecologic Oncology. 2008;**111**(1):41-45

[34] Bell MC et al. Comparison of outcomes and cost for endometrial cancer staging via traditional laparotomy, standard laparoscopy and robotic techniques. Gynecologic Oncology. 2008;**111**(3):407-411

[35] Lim PC, Kang E, Park DH. Learning curve and surgical outcome for robotic-assisted hysterectomy with lymphadenectomy: Case-matched controlled comparison with laparoscopy and laparotomy for treatment of endometrial cancer. Journal of Minimally Invasive Gynecology. 2010;**17**(6):739-748

[36] Magrina JF et al. Robotic surgery for endometrial cancer: Comparison of perioperative outcomes and recurrence with laparoscopy, vaginal/laparoscopy and laparotomy. European Journal of Gynaecological Oncology. 2011;**32**(5):476-480

[37] Seamon LG et al. Comprehensive surgical staging for endometrial cancer in obese patients: Comparing robotics and laparotomy. Obstetrics and Gynecology. 2009;**114**(1):16-21

[38] DeNardis SA et al. Robotically assisted laparoscopic hysterectomy versus total abdominal hysterectomy and lymphadenectomy for endometrial cancer. Gynecologic Oncology. 2008;**111**(3):412-417

[39] ElSahwi KS et al. Comparison between 155 cases of robotic vs. 150 cases of open surgical staging for endometrial cancer. Gynecologic Oncology. 2012;**124**(2):260-264

[40] Subramaniam A et al. A cohort study evaluating robotic versus laparotomy surgical outcomes of obese women with endometrial carcinoma. Gynecologic Oncology. 2011;**122**(3):604-607

[41] Barnett JC et al. Cost comparison among robotic, laparoscopic, and open hysterectomy for endometrial cancer. Obstetrics and Gynecology. 2010;**116**(3):685-693

[42] Boggess JF et al. A case-control study of robot-assisted type III radical hysterectomy with pelvic lymph node dissection compared with open radical hysterectomy. American Journal of Obstetrics and Gynecology. 2008;**199**(4):357e1-357e7

[43] Soliman PT et al. Radical hysterectomy: A comparison of surgical approaches after adoption of robotic surgery in gynecologic oncology. Gynecologic Oncology. 2011;**123**(2): 333-336

[44] Cantrell LA et al. Survival outcomes for women undergoing type III robotic radical hysterectomy for cervical cancer: A 3-year experience. Gynecologic Oncology. 2010;**117**(2): 260-265

[45] Geisler JP et al. Robotically assisted laparoscopic radical hysterectomy compared with open radical hysterectomy. International Journal of Gynecological Cancer. 2010;**20**(3): 438-442

[46] Nam EJ et al. A case-control study of robotic radical hysterectomy and pelvic lymphadenectomy using 3 robotic arms compared with abdominal radical hysterectomy in cervical cancer. International Journal of Gynecological Cancer. 2010;**20**(7):1284-1289

[47] Holloway RW et al. Comparison of total laparoscopic and abdominal radical hysterectomy for patients with early-stage cervical cancer. Obstetrics and Gynecology. 2007;**110**(5):1174, author reply 1174-5

[48] Magrina JF. Robotic surgery in gynecology. European Journal of Gynaecological Oncology. 2007;**28**(2):77-82

[49] Puntambekar SP et al. Laparoscopic total radical hysterectomy by the Pune technique: Our experience of 248 cases. Journal of Minimally Invasive Gynecology. 2007;**14**(6):682-689

[50] Obermair A et al. A phase III randomized clinical trial comparing laparoscopic or robotic radical hysterectomy with abdominal radical hysterectomy in patients with early stage cervical cancer. Journal of Minimally Invasive Gynecology. 2008;**15**(5):584-588

[51] Estape R et al. A case matched analysis of robotic radical hysterectomy with lymphadenectomy compared with laparoscopy and laparotomy. Gynecologic Oncology. 2009;**113**(3): 357-361

[52] Fanning J, Fenton B, Purohit M. Robotic radical hysterectomy. American Journal of Obstetrics and Gynecology. 2008;**198**(6):649e1-649e4

[53] Kim YT et al. Robotic radical hysterectomy with pelvic lymphadenectomy for cervical carcinoma: A pilot study. Gynecologic Oncology. 2008;**108**(2):312-316

[54] Maggioni A et al. Robotic approach for cervical cancer: Comparison with laparotomy: A case control study. Gynecologic Oncology. 2009;**115**(1):60-64

[55] Nezhat FR et al. Robotic radical hysterectomy versus total laparoscopic radical hysterectomy with pelvic lymphadenectomy for treatment of early cervical cancer. JSLS. 2008;**12**(3):227-237

[56] Persson J et al. Robot assisted laparoscopic radical hysterectomy and pelvic lymphadenectomy with short and long term morbidity data. Gynecologic Oncology. 2009;**113**(2): 185-190

[57] Sert BM, Abeler VM. Robotic-assisted laparoscopic radical hysterectomy (Piver type III) with pelvic node dissection—Case report. European Journal of Gynaecological Oncology. 2006;**27**(5):531-533

[58] Sert B, Abeler V. Robotic radical hysterectomy in early-stage cervical carcinoma patients, comparing results with total laparoscopic radical hysterectomy cases. The future is now? International Journal of Medical Robotics. 2007;**3**(**3**):224-228

[59] Field JB et al. Computer-enhanced robotic surgery in gynecologic oncology. Surgical Endoscopy. 2007;**21**(2):244-246

[60] Kho RM et al. Robotic hysterectomy: Technique and initial outcomes. American Journal of Obstetrics and Gynecology. 2007;**197**(1):113e1-113e4

[61] van Dam PA et al. Robotic-assisted laparoscopic cytoreductive surgery for lobular carcinoma of the breast metastatic to the ovaries. Journal of Minimally Invasive Gynecology. 2007;**14**(6):746-749

[62] Bandera CA, Magrina JF. Robotic surgery in gynecologic oncology. Current Opinion in Obstetrics & Gynecology. 2009;**21**(1):25-30

[63] Choi SB et al. Early experiences of robotic-assisted laparoscopic liver resection. Yonsei Medical Journal. 2008;**49**(4):632-638

[64] Nadeem R, Abu-Rustum RRB, Douglas A. Levine, Atlas of Procedures in Gynecologic Oncology. 3rd ed. CRC Press Taylor and Francis Group, Third Edition; 2013. p. 472

[65] Jung YW et al. The feasibility of scarless single-port transumbilical total laparoscopic hysterectomy: Initial clinical experience. Surgical Endoscopy. 2010;**24**(7):1686-1692

[66] Kim YW et al. Single-port laparoscopic myomectomy using a new single-port transumbilical morcellation system: Initial clinical study. Journal of Minimally Invasive Gynecology. 2010;**17**(5):587-592

[67] Kim TJ et al. Single port access laparoscopic adnexal surgery. Journal of Minimally Invasive Gynecology. 2009;**16**(5):612-615

[68] Ramirez PT. Single-port laparoscopic surgery: Is a single incision the next frontier in minimally invasive gynecologic surgery? Gynecologic Oncology. 2009;**114**(2):143-144

[69] Fader AN, Escobar PF. Laparoendoscopic single-site surgery (LESS) in gynecologic oncology: Technique and initial report. Gynecologic Oncology. 2009;**114**(2):157-161

[70] Paek J et al. Robotic single-site versus laparoendoscopic single-site hysterectomy: A propensity score matching study. Surgical Endoscopy. 2016;**30**(3):1043-1050

[71] Lopez S, Mulla Z, Hernandez L, Garza DM, Payne TN, Farnam RW. A comparison of outcomes between robotic-assisted, single-site laparoscopy versus laparoendoscopic single site for benign hysterectomy. Journal of Minimally Invasive Gynecology. 2016;**23**(1)

[72] Gungor M et al. Single-port hysterectomy: Robotic versus laparoscopic. Journal of Robotic Surgery. Mar 2018;**12**(1):87-92

[73] Buckley de Meritens A et al. Feasibility and learning curve of robotic laparoendoscopic single-site surgery in gynecology. Journal of Minimally Invasive Gynecology. 2017; **24**(2):323-328

[74] Manoucheri MAUDE: analysis of robotic-assisted gynecologic surgery. Journal of Minimally Invasive Gynecology. Jul-Aug 2014;**21**(4):592-595

[75] Tse KY et al. Robot-assisted gynaecological cancer surgery-complications and prevention. Best Practice and Research Clinical Obstretrics and Gynaecology. Nov 2017;**45**:94-106

[76] Park DA, Yun JE, Kim SW, et al. Surgical and clinical safety and effectiveness of robotassisted laparoscopic hysterectomy compared to conventional laparoscopy and laparotomy for cervical cancer: A systematic review and meta-analysis. European Journal of Surgical Oncology. Sep 2016;**42**(9):1303-14

[77] Merritt AJ, Crosbie EJ, Charova J, et al. Prophylactic pre-operative bilateral ureteric catheters for major gynaecological surgery. Archives of Gynecology and Obstetrics. 2013;**288**:1061-1066

[78] Han L, Cao R, Jiang JY, et al. Preset ureter catheter in laparoscopic radical hysterectomy of cervical cancer. Genetics and Molecular Research. 2014;**13**:3638-3645

[79] Picerno T, Sloan NL, Escobar P, et al. Bowel injury in robotic gynecologic surgery: Risk factors and management options. A systematic review. American Journal of Obstetrics and Gynecology. 2017;**216**:10-26

[80] Landeen LB, Hultgren EM, Kapsch TM, Mallory PW. Vaginal cuff dehiscence: A randomized trial comparing robotic vaginal cuff closure methods. Journal of Robotic Surgery. 2016;**10**(4):337-341

[81] Drudi L, Press JZ, Lau S, et al. Vaginal vault dehiscence after robotic hysterectomy for gynecologic cancers: Search for risk factors and literature review. International Journal of Gynecological Cancer. 2013;**23**:943-950

[82] Shields K, Minion L, Sumner D, Monk B. Ten year food and drug administration reporting of robot-assisted laparoscopy complications, deaths, and device malfunctions in gynecologic surgery. Gynecologic Oncology. 2014;**135**(2):402. DOI: 10.1016/j.ygyno.2014.07.061

Chapter 4

Laparoscopic Surgery for Gastric Cancer

Talha Sarigoz, Inanc Samil Sarici, Ozgul Duzgun and Mustafa Uygar Kalayci

Additional information is available at the end of the chapter

http://dx.doi.org/10.5772/intechopen.72852

Abstract

In patients with gastric cancer, surgical resection is the only treatment that can offer cure or increase long-term survival. With the accumulation of experience in laparoscopic radical gastrectomy and the progress in surgical instruments, laparoscopic surgery for gastric cancer has gained popularity despite initial concerns regarding safety and oncological adequacy. As a result, laparoscopic technique has been widely applied in gastric cancer. Different meta-analyses showed that laparoscopic procedures are associated with less blood loss but longer operation time. Many studies have reported outcomes of laparoscopic surgery for early gastric cancer, but several authors also have shown that a laparoscopic approach can also be used in cases of advanced gastric cancer. We therefore conducted this study to expand our experience and to evaluate laparoscopic gastrectomy step by step in the light of recent reports while defining key points and surgical technique.

Keywords: laparoscopic surgery, gastric cancer, gastrectomy, lymphadenectomy, advanced, early gastric cancer, laparoscopic gastrectomy

1. Introduction

Gastric cancer (GC) is the fifth most common malignancy and the third most common cause of cancer-related deaths worldwide in both sexes combined [1]. Surgery with either total or subtotal gastrectomy and lymphadenectomy is the initial treatment [2]. The first example of gastrectomy for cancer was described by Theodor Billroth and the first laparoscopy-assisted gastrectomy was performed by Kitano et al. in 1991 for a patient with early GC [3, 4]. In the last two decades, in parallel to advances in surgical devices and technical expertise, minimally invasive surgery has become the new trend and the laparoscopy has increasingly started being applied for GC as an alternative to open surgery. However, due to complexity of the lymph node structure and contiguity of stomach to gross vascular structures, it is technically demanding. During the procedure, it is equally important to ensure adequate resection and pay attention to some precautions [5]. In this chapter, we will clarify pre-operative approach, technical considerations as well as clinical outcomes of laparoscopic surgery (LS) for GC based on the recent reports in the literature.

2. Preoperative approach

2.1. Indications for laparoscopic surgery

Most of the reports evaluated early GC population and common consensus is that laparoscopic gastrectomy is appropriate for early-stage GC with benefits of reduced need for painkillers, early discharge, rapid recovery of bowel movement, less pulmonary function disorders, and better cosmetic results [5, 6]. There is agreement about performing laparoscopic total gastrectomy for proximal GC with T1 N0 disease and laparoscopic distal gastrectomy for distal GC with T1–2 N0 disease [5]. Regarding advanced stage cancers, there is still debate over appropriateness of laparoscopy concerning oncologic adequacy of lymphadenectomy with tumor-free margins. Recent meta-analysis and cohorts demonstrated favorable short- and long-term outcomes of laparoscopic gastrectomy for advanced stage GC; but in order to recommend it as an alternative to open surgery, there is still room for prospective clinical trials and longer-follow-up studies [7–9].

2.2. Determination of resection margin

Lack of tactile feedback limits assessment of the tumor during laparoscopic surgery. Since laparoscopic gastrectomy has been performed mostly for early GC and achieving tumor-free margins is important in terms of oncological principles, different methods have been proposed for safe determination of resection line in tumors without serosal surface invasion. Reported various procedures include preoperative or intraoperative endoscopic dye injection, preoperative endoscopic clipping along with intraoperative endoscopy, intraoperative radiography or ultrasonography [10–14]. None of these methods has wide acceptance and choice of technique vary with institution.

2.3. Nutritional status of patients

As gastric cancer is a serious malignancy of the upper intestinal tract, patients are at risk for malnutrition due to maldigestion and malabsorption. On the other hand, surgery itself imposes protein and energy requirements and it can aggravate pre-existing nutritional disorders [15]. There is a lack of clinical evidence about role of laparoscopic gastrectomy in malnourished patients with GC. A recent retrospective study reported significantly less post-operative complications and faster recovery for laparoscopic gastrectomy compared to open surgery [16]. But, prospective clinical trials to analyze short- and long-term effects of pre-operative nutritional support, chemotherapy and dissection type are required to recommend laparoscopic gastrectomy for malnourished patients.

2.4. Presence of enlarged lymph nodes in preoperative imaging

There are controversies on the extent of lymphadenectomy for GC. Nevertheless, lymph node dissection is recommended for staging and prevention of local recurrence. Most of the patients with GC are diagnosed at a later stage of the disease, often with enlarged lymph nodes. Since lymphadenectomy is a challenging procedure, especially in laparoscopic setting, enlarged nodes interfere with anatomical structures and disrupt the course of the dissection. In a late retrospective study, performing laparoscopic gastrectomy for GC with pre-operative enlarged lymph nodes was found to be safe and effective [17]. Yet, these results should be supported with prospective research to make recommendation.

2.5. Obese patients

Obese patients carry high risk for comorbid diseases and they are directly associated with intra- and post-operative complications [18]. Obesity was considered as a relative contraindication for laparoscopy, but with the advances in laparoscopic equipment and growing experience, initial studies with laparoscopic surgery in obese patients have shown promise [19]. According to the reports in the literature, due to abundant visceral fat content and difficult manipulation of tissue, operation times in laparoscopic gastrectomy were longer compared to open surgery [20, 21]. Not only obesity, but also high body mass index (BMI ≥ 25 kg/m^2) was shown to affect operation time and retrieved lymph node number negatively [22]. On the other hand, the 5-year survival rates of patients who underwent laparoscopic gastrectomy and open gastrectomy were similar [23]. But regarding early post-operative outcomes, we cannot mention that there is an agreement [20, 21, 23]. Despite negative findings, laparoscopic gastrectomy is likely to be the choice of surgery in obese patients with growing experience.

2.6. Elderly patients

In parallel to increasing age, functional capacity decreases at some point and this situation creates risk for surgery. Considering advantages, elderly may benefit from laparoscopic surgery. In an updated pooled meta-analysis, laparoscopic gastrectomy was found to reduce surgery-related cardiopulmonary disease and also better cognitive outcomes were observed compared to open surgery [24]. But, lack of randomized controlled studies in the literature prevent from making precise conclusions.

3. Technical considerations

3.1. The importance of lymphadenectomy in gastric cancer

Lymph node metastasis (LNM) is the most common pattern of metastatic spread in gastric cancer [25]. The reported frequency of LNM in gastric cancer can be seen up to 80%. Lymphatic networks are plenty in the layer of the gastric wall, particularly in the submucosa and serosa, which simplify metastasis. Oncological outcomes will not be reached if gastrectomy alone is performed for gastric cancer. Therefore, lymphatic flow of the stomach and characteristics of metastasis have been continuously examined by researchers. In the Japanese gastric cancer treatment guidelines based on the third English edition of the Japanese Classification of Gastric Carcinoma and the Japanese Gastric Cancer Association defined the extent of systematic lymphadenectomy according to the type of gastrectomy indicated [26]. Lymph node metastasis in gastric cancer is usually associated with the location of the tumor, and metastasis follows the lymphatic drainage routes from the superficial to the profoundus. For this reason, lymph nodes are numbered and dissection for functional lymph node resection was defined. Laparoscopic gastrectomy, which begins with D1 dissection in early gastric cancer treatment, can now be done easily with the aid of technology (laparoscopy, robotic surgery) and D2 dissection technique is routinely performed in the treatment of advanced GC [27] (**Tables 1** and **2**).

3.2. Surgical technique of laparoscopic gastrectomy with D2 lymphadenectomy

3.2.1. Patient's position and location of trocars

The patient is placed in the modified lithotomy position. The surgical table is adjusted 20–30° into the reverse Trendelenburg position. The surgeon stands on the patient's leg, the assistant is on the right side, and the camera operator is between the patient's left side. Besides routine laparoscopic devices, advance vessel sealing systems, all types of intestinal Endo-GIA and circular staplers must be available on the operating table. The intervention generally performed by using five ports. Additionally, subxiphoid sixth port can be required during the splenic hilar lymph node dissection. 10-mm optic port is placed 1 cm above the umbilicus. 15-mm trocar left preaxillary and 5 mm trocar right preaxillary is inserted in the line 2 cm below the costal margin. Two 5-mm ports are placed bilaterally in each hypochondrium for assisting and dissection purposes (**Figure 1**).

3.2.2. Surgical procedure

Laparoscopic exploration is used for preoperative staging, liver and peritoneal metastasis which can reduce unnecessary laparotomies. Once it is determined that it is suitable for surgery, the procedure continues in four steps as left part region, right part region, cardiac region, and reconstruction (**Table 3**).

3.2.2.1. Left part region (4sa, 4sv, 10, 11d)

The approach for removing the greater omentum begins from the superior border of the transverse colon. After that, the division is extended toward the flexura of left and the right colon. In the continuation of the dissection, splenic ligaments must be separated due to prevent of iatrogenic splenic injury which may be caused by traction. Gastrosplenic, splenocolic, splenorenal, and splenophrenic ligaments need to be separated in this stage. The omentectomy helps to achieve a lymphadenectomy corresponding to lymph node stations 4sa and 4sv according to the Japanese classification. The left gastro-omental vessels are perfectly identified clipped and divided. After this dissection, the short gastric vessels will be divided using the sealing

http://dx.doi.org/10.5772/intechopen.72852

Regional lymph nodes of stomach
1. Right cardia lymph nodes
2. Left cardia lymph nodes
3. Lymph nodes along the lesser curvature
4. Lymph nodes along the greater curvature
• Station **4sa:** lymph nodes along the short gastric vessels
• Station **4sb:** lymph nodes along the left gastroepiploic vessels
• Station **4d:** lymph nodes along the right gastroepiploic vessel
5. Suprapyloric group of lymph nodes or nodes along the right gastric artery
6. Infrapyloric groups of lymph nodes
7. Lymph nodes along the left gastric artery
8. Lymph nodes along the common hepatic artery
• Station **8a:** anterosuperior group
• Station **8b:** posterior group
9. Lymph nodes around the celiac artery
10. Lymph nodes at the splenic hilum
11. Lymph nodes along the splenic artery
• Station **11p:** along the proximal splenic artery
• Station **11d:** along the distal splenic artery
12. Lymph nodes in the hepatoduodenal ligament
• Station **12a:** along the hepatic artery
• Station **12b:** along the bile duct
• Station **12p**: behind the portal vein
13. Lymph nodes behind the pancreatic head
14. Lymph nodes at the root of the mesentery or the SMA
15. Lymph nodes along the middle colic artery
16. Para-aortic group of lymph nodes
• Station **16a1:** lymph node in the aortic hiatus
• Station **16a2:** lymph node around the abdominal aorta (from the upper margin of the celiac trunk to the lower margin of the left renal vein)
• Station **16b1:** lymph node around the abdominal aorta (from the lower margin of the left renal vein to the upper margin of the inferior mesenteric artery)
• Station **16b2:** lymph node around the abdominal aorta (from the upper margin of the inferior mesenteric artery to the aortic bifurcation)

Table 1. Numbering lymph nodes according to the Japanese Research Society for Gastric Cancer.

D0	No dissection or incomplete dissection of the Group 1 nodes
D1	Dissection of all the Group 1 nodes (No.1–6 lymph nodes)
D2	Dissection of all the Group 1 and Group 2 nodes (D1 station + No.7–11 lymph nodes)
D3	Dissection of all the Group 1, Group 2 and Group 3 nodes (D2+ No. 12–16 lymph nodes)

Table 2. Definitions of lymphadenectomy in gastric cancer.

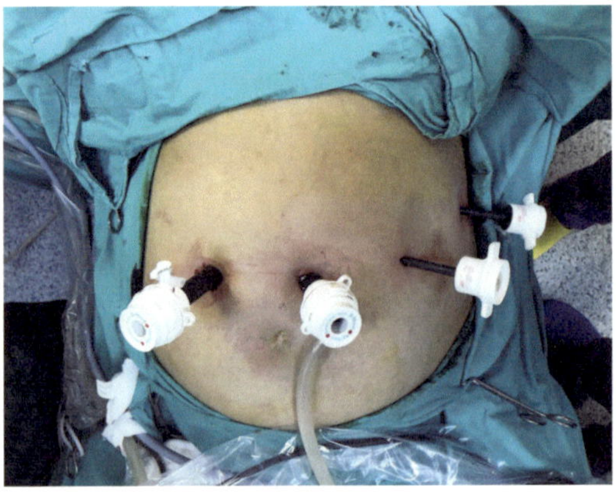

Figure 1. Patient's position and location of trocars.

1	Left part region (4sa, 4sv, 10, 11d)
2	Right part region (4d, 5, 6, 7, 8a, 8p, 9, 11p, 12a, 12b, 12p)
3	Cardiac region [1–3]
4	Gastric resection and reconstruction

Table 3. Steps of laparoscopic gastrectomy for gastric cancer.

systems. This dissection should be continued until the left crus of the diaphragm clearly seen. At this time, the lymph node 10 and 11d in the splenic hilus is gently excised (**Figures 2** and **3**).

3.2.2.2. Right part region (4d, 5, 6, 7, 8a, 8p, 9, 11p, 12a, 12b, 12p)

The dissection is then continued toward the right part of the abdomen. Dissection of the gastro-omental ligament is pursued in this area. This dissection allows to drop the right colon and to access the duodenum. This maneuver also allows to expose the anterior aspect of the pancreatic head and to access the right gastro-omental pedicle, where a lymphadenectomy should be performed in order to control lymph node station 6 (**Figure 4**).

Right gastro-omental vessels are dissected, isolated, and divided. Once this first mobilization and 6-station of lymphadenectomy step has been performed, the first portion of the duodenum will be dissected and isolated, prior to moving on to the supragastric compartment. The common bile duct, hepatic artery, and portal vein, which form the hepatoduodenal ligament,

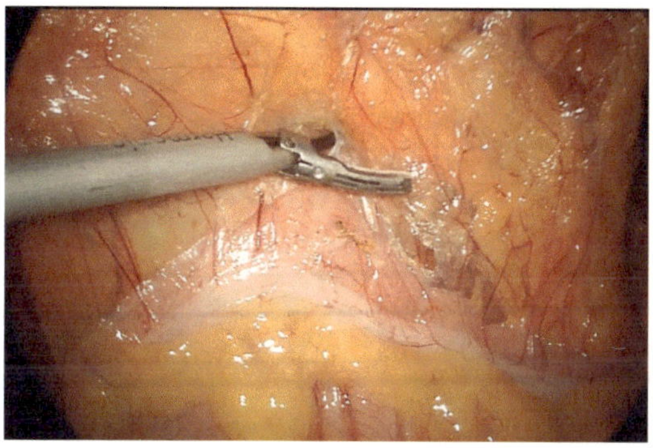

Figure 2. Lift of transvers colon and dissection of anterior transvers mesocolon fascia.

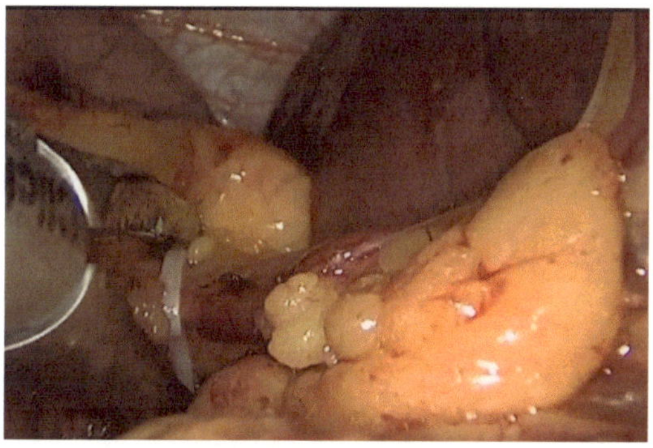

Figure 3. The left gastro-omental vessel is clipped and divided.

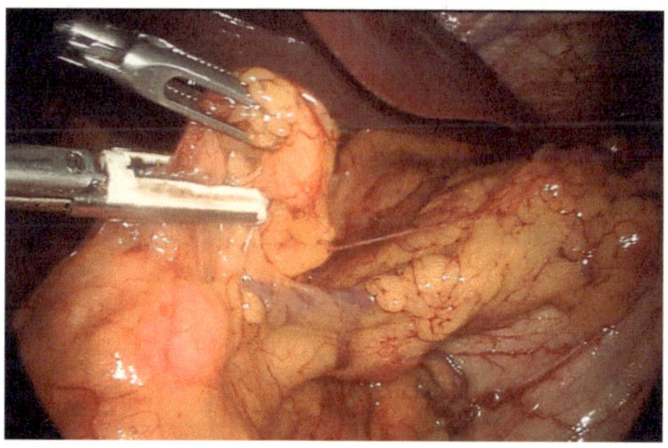

Figure 4. Dissection of number 6 lymphatic area.

are identified. The right gastric artery will also be identified and divided along with lymph node dissection at the level of lymph node station 5. The 12a, 12b, and 12p lymph node stations in the hepatoduodenal ligament are excised with vessel sealing devices (**Figure 5**).

Duodenal division is then performed approximately 2 cm distally from the pylorus by Endo-GIA blue cartridge. After dissection of the hepatic proper artery, resection will be carried on at the superior border of the pancreas at the level of the common hepatic artery, namely lymph node

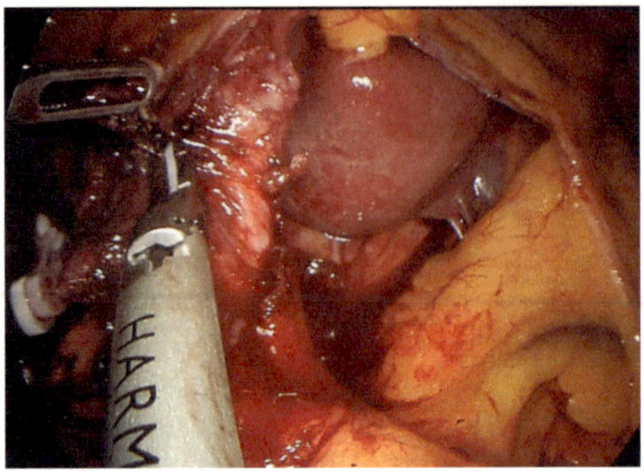

Figure 5. Dissection of hepatoduodenal lymphatic area.

stations 8 and 9. The left coronary vein is also identified, clipped, and divided. Dissection is pursued toward the coeliac trunk with lymph node dissection of stations 9. Dissection of the left gastric artery is begun along with lymph node dissection of station 7. The left gastric artery is clipped and divided. After that 11p lymph node stations along the splenic artery are excised. Care should be taken during dissection due to the tortuous structure of splenic artery (**Figures 6** and **7**).

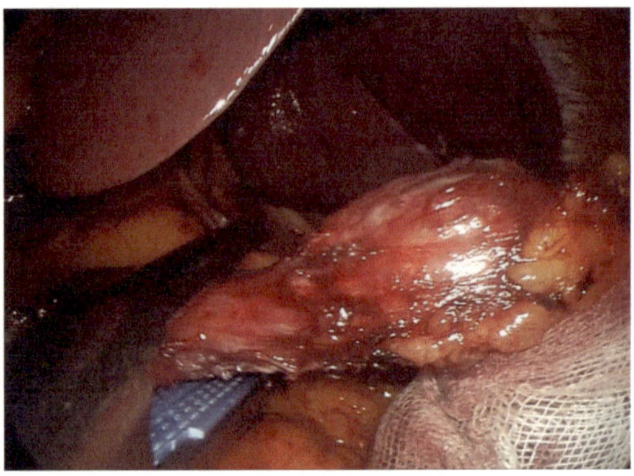

Figure 6. Transection of duodenum.

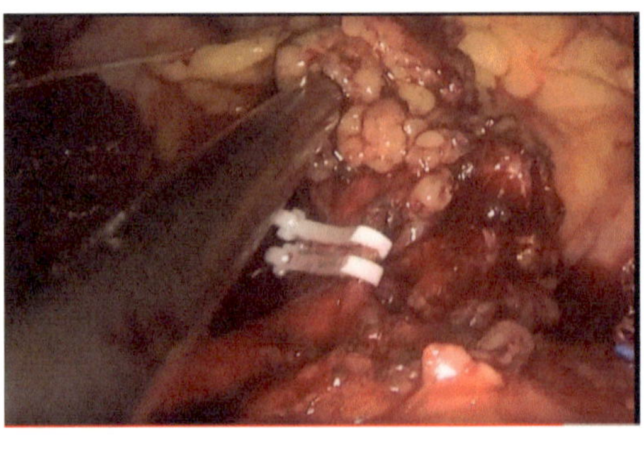

Figure 7. Dissection of number 7, 8, and 9 lymphatic area.

3.2.2.3. Cardiac region

The lymph nodes in the cardiac region are located on both sides of the cardia and along the lesser curvature [1–3]. Hepatogastric ligament is opened by vessel sealing devices in the avascular area at the posterior wall of the gastric lesser curvature. Thus, the gastric lesser curvature is fully bared and dissection of the No. 3 lymph nodes is done. The left and right diaphragm crus are identified and the phrenoesophageal membrane is dissected. Lymph nodes No:1 and No:2 are excised. The abdominal part of the esophagus is bared 5 cm in the abdomen. Left and right vagal nerves divided (**Figure 8**).

3.2.2.4. Gastric resection and reconstruction

The reconstruction should be in different forms according to the extent of the resection. Proximal resection was performed with Endo GIA blue cartridge which is placed from 15 mm trocar. Trans oral OrVil™ (Covidien Mansfield, USA) is propagated from the esophagus and anvil is placed in the esophageal stump. Transvers mesocolon lifted and the small window open from the avascular area. Jejunal ans is divided at 20 cm from the Treitz ligament by Endo GIA blue cartridge. Esophagojejunostomy is done with 25 mm circular stapler if totally gastrectomy planned or gastrojejunostomy is performed with EndoGIA if subtotal gastrectomy intended. Jejunal stump is closed with Endo GIA blue cartridge. Laparoscopic reinforcement

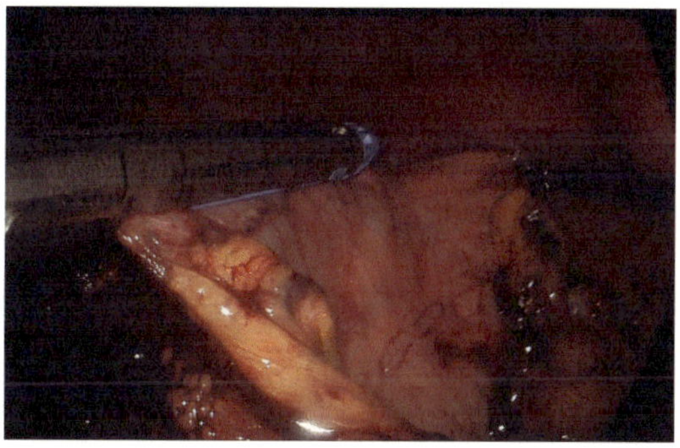

Figure 8. Dissection of cardiac lymphatic area.

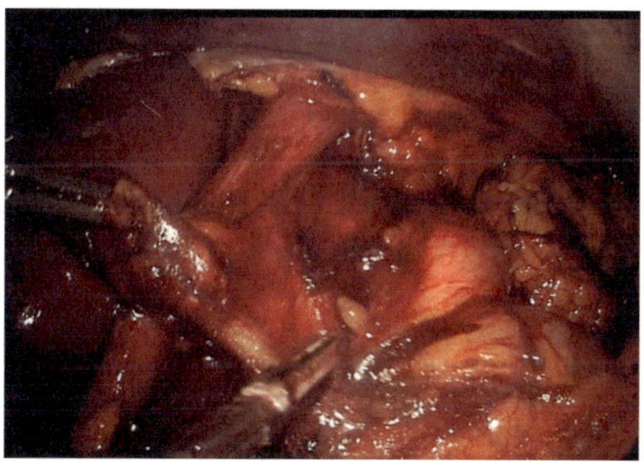

Figure 9. Proximal resection of stomach with EndoGIA.

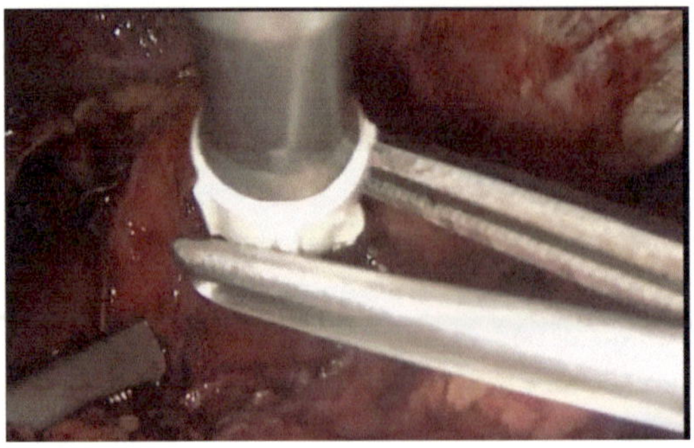

Figure 10. OrVil™ placement in the esophageal stump.

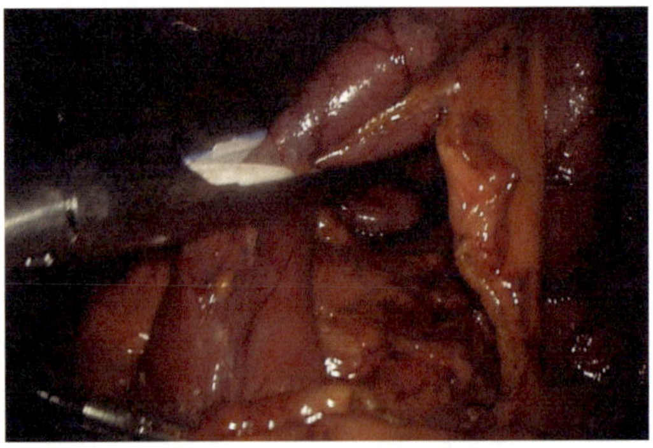

Figure 11. Division of jejunal ans 20 cm distal to the Treitz ligament.

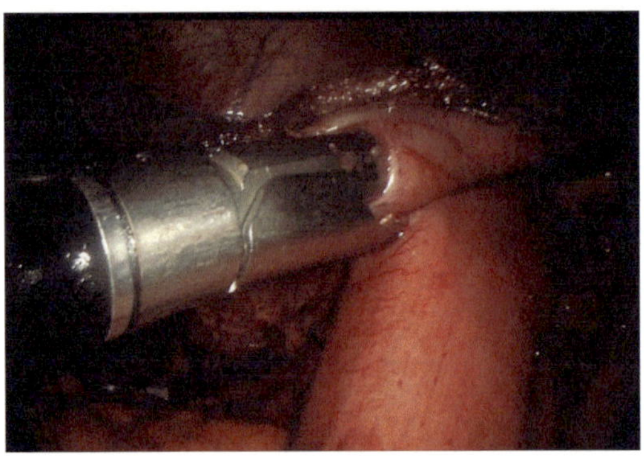

Figure 12. Gastrojejunostomy with EndoGIA.

sutures can be added if needed. Jejunum is fixed to the diaphragm crus. The jejunojejunostomy is also performed by means of a side to side Endo GIA blue cartridge stapler. Placement of the gastric tube is controlled laparoscopically. This tube is lowered until the distal part of the alimentary limb. A wound protector is placed into the defect, hence allowing for the extraction of the entire specimen, including the whole stomach and the omentum (**Figures 9–13**, **Table 4**).

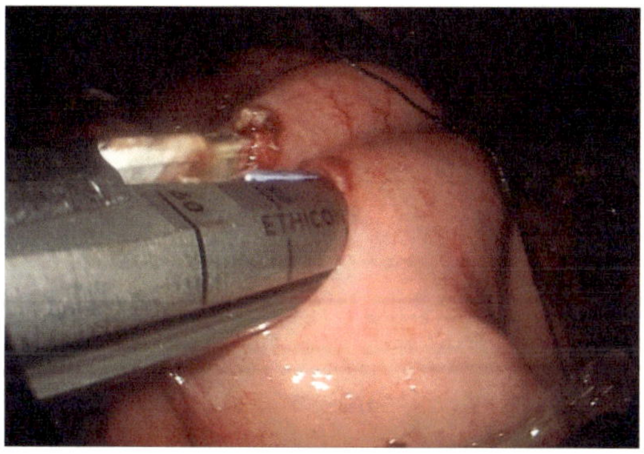

Figure 13. Jejunojejunostomy with EndoGIA.

Subtotal gastrectomy	Total gastrectomy

• Totally laparoscopic gastroduodenostomy (Billroth 1)
• Billroth 1 through mini laparotomy
• Billroth 1 with hand port
• Roux-en-Y Gastrojejunostomy
	• Roux-en-Y esophagojejunostomy
	• Hand-sewn anastomosis
	  • Laparoscopic
	  • Mini-laparotomy
	• Mechanical anastomosis
	  • Circular stapler
	  • Manually loaded anvil
	  • Transoral (OrVil™)

Table 4. Different reconstruction forms according to the resection types.

4. Post-operative outcomes

4.1. Early post-operative outcomes

Initial studies with laparoscopic gastrectomy consisted of mostly early GC and with growing experience it has been started to apply to later stages of the disease. Laparoscopic gastrectomy whether performed for early or advanced GC has advantages such as less blood loss, early ambulation, rapid recovery of bowel movement, and shorter hospitalization compared to open surgery [28–31]. Complication rates of laparoscopic gastrectomy for early GC ranged from 4.2 to 23.3% and these results did not differ from open surgery [29, 32–34]. In the latest ongoing clinical trials, short-term results have been shared. While, laparoscopic surgery for advanced GC has a complication rate of 16.4%, it is 24.3% for open surgery [35–37]. These studies will be finalized in 2018. In an ongoing study in Japan, short-term results have revealed incidence of anastomotic leakage rate as 4.7% for laparoscopic surgery in advanced stage [37]. In the retrospective studies, anastomotic leakage rate during LS for advanced GC was reported to range from 1.1 to 2.7% [30, 38–40]. But this risk should be evaluated appropriately.

4.2. Late post-operative outcomes

According to single-center studies, after laparoscopic gastrectomy for early GC, the morbidity rates ranged from 10 to 14.8% and mortality rates from 0 to 1.1% [6, 41, 42]. Regarding laparoscopic gastrectomy for AGC, the morbidity rates ranged from 8.0 to 24.2% but there was no significant difference compared to open surgery [30, 39, 40]. There are ongoing randomized phase-II and III studies in Asian Countries. They are expected to give scientifically more reliable results [30, 35]. Initial results indicate that LS for advanced GC is feasible and safe but surgeon experience and institution volume play important role on patient outcome. Long-term outcomes should be clarified with well-established studies.

Author details

Talha Sarigoz[1]*, Inanc Samil Sarici[2], Ozgul Duzgun[3] and Mustafa Uygar Kalayci[4]

*Address all correspondence to: sarigozt.md@gmail.com

1 Department of General Surgery, Sason State Hospital, Batman, Turkey

2 Department of General Surgery, Kanuni Sultan Suleyman Training and Research Hospital, Istanbul, Turkey

3 Division of Surgical Oncology, Department of General Surgery, Umraniye Training and Research Hospital, Istanbul, Turkey

4 Department of General Surgery, Kanuni Sultan Suleyman Training and Research Hospital, Istanbul, Turkey

References

[1] Global Burden of Disease Cancer C, Fitzmaurice C, Allen C, Barber RM, Barregard L, Bhutta ZA, et al. Global, regional, and national cancer incidence, mortality, years of life lost, years lived with disability, and disability-adjusted life-years for 32 cancer groups, 1990 to 2015: A systematic analysis for the global burden of disease study. JAMA Oncology. 2017;**3**(4):524-548

[2] Lutz MP, Zalcberg JR, Ducreux M, Ajani JA, Allum W, Aust D, et al. Highlights of the EORTC St. Gallen International Expert Consensus on the primary therapy of gastric, gastroesophageal and oesophageal cancer—Differential treatment strategies for subtypes of early gastroesophageal cancer. European Journal of Cancer. 2012;**48**(16):2941-2953

[3] Kitano S, Iso Y, Moriyama M, Sugimachi K. Laparoscopy-assisted Billroth I Gastrectomy. Surgical Laparoscopy & Endoscopy. 1994;**4**(2):146-148

[4] Billroth T. Offenes schreiben an Herr, Dr. L. Wittelshofer. Wiener Medizinische Wochenschrift. 1881;**26**:731

[5] Brar S, Law C, McLeod R, Helyer L, Swallow C, Paszat L, et al. Defining surgical quality in gastric cancer: A RAND/UCLA appropriateness study. Journal of the American College of Surgeons. 2013;**217**(2):347-357. e1

[6] Kitano S, Shiraishi N, Fujii K, Yasuda K, Inomata M, Adachi YA. Randomized controlled trial comparing open vs laparoscopy-assisted distal gastrectomy for the treatment of early gastric cancer: An interim report. Surgery. 2002;**131**(1 Suppl):S306-S311

[7] Son T, Hyung WJ, Lee JH, Kim YM, Noh SH. Minimally invasive surgery for serosa-positive gastric cancer (pT4a) in patients with preoperative diagnosis of cancer without serosal invasion. Surgical Endoscopy. 2014;**28**(3):866-874

[8] Lee J, Kim W. Long-term outcomes after laparoscopy-assisted gastrectomy for advanced gastric cancer: Analysis of consecutive 106 experiences. Journal of Surgical Oncology. 2009;**100**(8):693-698

[9] Huscher CG, Mingoli A, Sgarzini G, Brachini G, Binda B, Di Paola M, et al. Totally laparoscopic total and subtotal gastrectomy with extended lymph node dissection for early and advanced gastric cancer: Early and long-term results of a 100-patient series. American Journal of Surgery. 2007;**194**(6):839-844. discussion 44

[10] Xuan Y, Hur H, Byun CS, Han SU, Cho YK. Efficacy of intraoperative gastroscopy for tumor localization in totally laparoscopic distal gastrectomy for cancer in the middle third of the stomach. Surgical Endoscopy. 2013;**27**(11):4364-4370

[11] Park DJ, Lee HJ, Kim SG, Jung HC, Song IS, Lee KU, et al. Intraoperative gastroscopy for gastric surgery. Surgical Endoscopy. 2005;**19**(10):1358-1361

[12] Nakagawa M, Ehara K, Ueno M, Tanaka T, Kaida S, Udagawa H. Accurate, safe, and rapid method of intraoperative tumor identification for totally laparoscopic distal gastrectomy: Injection of mixed fluid of sodium hyaluronate and patent blue. Surgical Endoscopy. 2014;**28**(4):1371-1375

[13] Kim HI, Hyung WJ, Lee CR, Lim JS, An JY, Cheong JH, et al. Intraoperative portable abdominal radiograph for tumor localization: A simple and accurate method for laparoscopic gastrectomy. Surgical Endoscopy. 2011;**25**(3):958-963

[14] Kawakatsu S, Ohashi M, Hiki N, Nunobe S, Nagino M, Sano T. Use of endoscopy to determine the resection margin during laparoscopic gastrectomy for cancer. The British Journal of Surgery. 2017

[15] Mariette C, De Botton ML, Piessen G. Surgery in esophageal and gastric cancer patients: What is the role for nutrition support in your daily practice? Annals of Surgical Oncology. 2012;**19**(7):2128-2134

[16] Zheng HL, Lu J, Zheng CH, Li P, Xie JW, Wang JB, et al. Short- and long-term outcomes in malnourished patients after laparoscopic or open radical gastrectomy. World Journal of Surgery. 2017

[17] Chen QY, Huang CM, Zheng CH, Li P, Xie JW, Wang JB, et al. Do preoperative enlarged lymph nodes affect the oncologic outcome of laparoscopic radical gastrectomy for gastric cancer? Oncotarget. 2017;**8**(5):8825-8834

[18] Tjeertes EK, Hoeks SE, Beks SB, Valentijn TM, Hoofwijk AG, Stolker RJ. Obesity—A risk factor for postoperative complications in general surgery? BMC Anesthesiology. 2015;**15**:112

[19] Loffer FD, Pent D. Laparoscopy in the obese patient. American Journal of Obstetrics and Gynecology. 1976;**125**(1):104-107

[20] Yasuda K, Inomata M, Shiraishi N, Izumi K, Ishikawa K, Kitano S. Laparoscopy-assisted distal gastrectomy for early gastric cancer in obese and nonobese patients. Surgical Endoscopy. 2004;**18**(8):1253-1256

[21] Kim MG, Yook JH, Kim KC, Kim TH, Kim HS, Kim BS, et al. Influence of obesity on early surgical outcomes of laparoscopic-assisted gastrectomy in gastric cancer. Surgical Laparoscopy, Endoscopy & Percutaneous Techniques. 2011;**21**(3):151-154

[22] Lee HJ, Kim HH, Kim MC, Ryu SY, Kim W, Song KY, et al. The impact of a high body mass index on laparoscopy assisted gastrectomy for gastric cancer. Surgical Endoscopy. 2009;**23**(11):2473-2479

[23] Son SY, Jung DH, Lee CM, Ahn SH, Ahn HS, Park DJ, et al. Laparoscopic gastrectomy versus open gastrectomy for gastric cancer in patients with body mass index of 30 kg/m^2 or more. Surgical Endoscopy. 2015;**29**(8):2126-2132

[24] Zong L, Wu A, Wang W, Deng J, Aikou S, Yamashita H, et al. Feasibility of laparoscopic gastrectomy for elderly gastric cancer patients: Meta-analysis of non-randomized controlled studies. Oncotarget. 2017;**8**(31):51878-51887

[25] Huang C-M, Zheng C-H. Summary of anatomy and physiology of perigastric lymphatic system. In: Huang C-M, Zheng C-H, editors. Laparoscopic Gastrectomy for Gastric Cancer: Surgical Technique and Lymphadenectomy. Dordrecht: Springer Netherlands; 2015. pp. 1-6

[26] Japanese Gastric Cancer A. Japanese gastric cancer treatment guidelines 2010 (ver. 3). Gastric Cancer. 2011;**14**(2):113-123

[27] RH T, Li P, Xie JW, Wang JB, Lin JX, Lu J, et al. Development of lymph node dissection in laparoscopic gastrectomy: Safety and technical tips. Transl. Gastroenterología y Hepatología. 2017;**2**:23

[28] Kim YW, Baik YH, Yun YH, Nam BH, Kim DH, Choi IJ, et al. Improved quality of life outcomes after laparoscopy-assisted distal gastrectomy for early gastric cancer: Results of a prospective randomized clinical trial. Annals of Surgery. 2008;**248**(5):721-727

[29] Kim HH, Hyung WJ, Cho GS, Kim MC, Han SU, Kim W, et al. Morbidity and mortality of laparoscopic gastrectomy versus open gastrectomy for gastric cancer: An interim report—A phase III multicenter, prospective, randomized trial (KLASS trial). Annals of Surgery. 2010;**251**(3):417-420

[30] Hu Y, Huang C, Sun Y, Su X, Cao H, Hu J, et al. Morbidity and mortality of laparoscopic versus open D2 distal Gastrectomy for advanced gastric cancer: A randomized controlled trial. Journal of Clinical Oncology. 2016;**34**(12):1350-1357

[31] Hayashi H, Ochiai T, Shimada H, Gunji Y. Prospective randomized study of open versus laparoscopy-assisted distal gastrectomy with extraperigastric lymph node dissection for early gastric cancer. Surgical Endoscopy. 2005;**19**(9):1172-1176

[32] Lee JH, Han HS, Lee JHA. Prospective randomized study comparing open vs laparoscopy-assisted distal gastrectomy in early gastric cancer: Early results. Surgical Endoscopy. 2005;**19**(2):168-173

[33] Hosono S, Arimoto Y, Ohtani H, Kanamiya Y. Meta-analysis of short-term outcomes after laparoscopy-assisted distal gastrectomy. World Journal of Gastroenterology. 2006; **12**(47):7676-7683

[34] Adachi Y, Shiraishi N, Shiromizu A, Bandoh T, Aramaki M, Kitano S. Laparoscopy-assisted Billroth I gastrectomy compared with conventional open gastrectomy. Archives of Surgery. 2000;**135**(7):806-810

[35] Lee H-J, Hyung WJ, Yang H-K, Han SU, Park Y-K, An JY, et al. Morbidity of laparoscopic distal gastrectomy with D2 lymphadenectomy compared with open distal gastrectomy for locally advanced gastric cancer: Short term outcomes from multicenter randomized controlled trial (KLASS-02). Journal of Clinical Oncology. 2016;**34**(15_suppl):4062

[36] Kinoshita T, Kaito A. Current status and future perspectives of laparoscopic radical surgery for advanced gastric cancer. Transl. Gastroenterología y Hepatología. 2017;**2**:43

[37] Inaki N, Etoh T, Ohyama T, Uchiyama K, Katada N, Koeda K, et al. A multi-institutional, prospective, phase II feasibility study of laparoscopy-assisted distal gastrectomy with D2 lymph node dissection for locally advanced gastric cancer (JLSSG0901). World Journal of Surgery. 2015;**39**(11):2734-2741

[38] Kim W, Song KY, Lee HJ, Han SU, Hyung WJ, Cho GS. The impact of comorbidity on surgical outcomes in laparoscopy-assisted distal gastrectomy: A retrospective analysis of multicenter results. Annals of Surgery. 2008;**248**(5):793-799

[39] Shinohara T, Satoh S, Kanaya S, Ishida Y, Taniguchi K, Isogaki J, et al. Laparoscopic versus open D2 gastrectomy for advanced gastric cancer: A retrospective cohort study. Surgical Endoscopy. 2013;**27**(1):286-294

[40] Park DJ, Han SU, Hyung WJ, Kim MC, Kim W, Ryu SY, et al. Long-term outcomes after laparoscopy-assisted gastrectomy for advanced gastric cancer: A large-scale multicenter retrospective study. Surgical Endoscopy. 2012;**26**(6):1548-1553

[41] Kitano S, Shiraishi N, Uyama I, Sugihara K, Tanigawa N, Japanese Laparoscopic Surgery Study Group. A multicenter study on oncologic outcome of laparoscopic gastrectomy for early cancer in Japan. Annals of Surgery. 2007;**245**(1):68-72

[42] Kim MC, Kim W, Kim HH, Ryu SW, Ryu SY, Song KY, et al. Risk factors associated with complication following laparoscopy-assisted Gastrectomy for gastric cancer: A large-scale Korean multicenter study. Annals of Surgical Oncology. 2008;**15**(10):2692-2700

Chapter 5

Total Laparoscopic Hysterectomy

Nidhi Sharma and Vanusha Selvin

Additional information is available at the end of the chapter

http://dx.doi.org/10.5772/intechopen.75652

Abstract

The applications of minimally invasive pelvic surgery continue to grow. This chapter focuses primarily on the preoperative evaluation, surgical technique and post-operative care of total laparoscopic hysterectomy. Since laparoscopic assisted vaginal hysterectomy is a slight modification of the procedure it is not being discussed separately. The major physiologic obstacles to safe laparoscopy include pregnancy, increased intra cranial pressure, abnormalities of cardiac output and gaseous exchange in the lung, chronic liver diseases and coagulation disorders. In a redo surgery there may be problems of laparoscopic port entry.

Keywords: hysterectomy, laparoscopy, surgery, total laparoscopic hysterectomy, laparoscopic supracervical hysterectomy, minimally invasive gynecological procedure

1. Introduction

The invention of Veress needle by Sir Janos Veres, an internist working in Hungary on tuberculosis, launched the era of laparoscopy [1]. The first laparoscopic hysterectomy was performed by Reich in 1989 [2]. Laparoscopic hysterectomy carries an edge over open hysterectomy as it provides a better magnification of anatomy and pathology [3–6].

The three main considerations are ergonomics, task analysis and minimizing injury and adhesions. When we apply the baseball diamond concept of trocar placement, the target in total laparoscopic hysterectomy is the uterine artery.

2. Preoperative evaluation

The goal of preoperative evaluation is to identify and modify risk factors that might adversely affect anesthetic care and surgical outcome.

2.1. History

1. Pulmonary disease—either obstructive or restrictive lung disease.
2. Cardiac disease
3. History of previous abdominal surgeries
4. History of coagulation disorders in self or in family
5. Previous history of anesthesia related complications
6. History of dentures or prosthetic devices
7. Previous operative records if any

2.2. Physical examination

1. Assessment of head and neck
2. Assessment of lungs and heart
3. Vascular and neurological examination
4. Airway evaluation by anesthetist
5. Vital signs
6. Abdominal examination to look for scar site and to decide on alternate port site and to assess the extent of adhesions.

2.3. Basic prerequisites before laparoscopic surgery

1. Hemoglobin
2. Blood urea and creatinine
3. Serum electrolytes
4. Liver function test
5. Coagulation profile
6. ECG and chest X-ray
7. Serology testing
8. Ultrasound abdomen and pelvis
9. Urine analysis

http://dx.doi.org/10.5772/intechopen.75652

Tests obtained within 6 months of surgery are acceptable if there is no significant change in patient medical history.

2.4. Patient education

The expectations with regard to the surgery should be clearly discussed with the patient. Anesthetic and surgical procedure and complications should be clearly explained to the patient. Risk of perioperative morbidity and mortality, post op pain, recovery, length of stay everything in detail should be counseled to the patient prior to surgery. Detailed informed consent regarding chance of conversion to laparotomy, chance of visceral injury should be obtained.

3. Surgical technique

The laparoscopic hysterectomy is classified depending on the extent of dissection done laparoscopically (**Table 1**). The knowledge of anatomy is essential before hysterectomy (**Figure 1**). The sterile precautions are maintained to arrange and assemble the laparoscopy instruments (**Figure 2**).

3.1. Positioning

The patient is given general anesthesia, with oral tracheal intubation. The patient is positioned in dorsal decubitus position Loyd Davis Position. The legs are positioned in the low lithotomy position with thighs flexed at 30°and knees supported, the arms are positioned along the body, and the buttocks extending slightly over the edge of the surgical table. The bladder is catheterized. The surgeon is positioned to the left of the patient. The first assistant

Hysterectomy Type	Description
I	Diagnostic laparoscopy and vaginal hysterectomy
II	Laparoscopic assisted vaginal Hysterectomy
III	Laparoscopic hysterectomy
IV	Total Laparoscopic Hysterectomy
V	Laparoscopic supracervical Hysterectomy
VI	Vaginal Hysterectomy with Laparoscopic Vault suspension
VII	Laparoscopic Hysterectomy with lymphadenectomy
VIII	Laparoscopic hysterectomy with lymphadenectomy and omentectomy
IX	Laparoscopic radical hysterectomy and lymphadenectomy

Table 1. The classification of laparoscopy assisted hysterectomy.

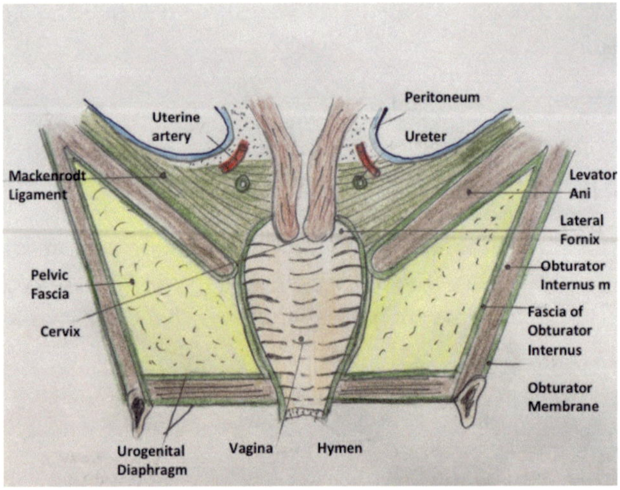

Figure 1. A sagittal section of a cadaveric specimen of female pelvis showing the anterior and posterior relation of the uterus.

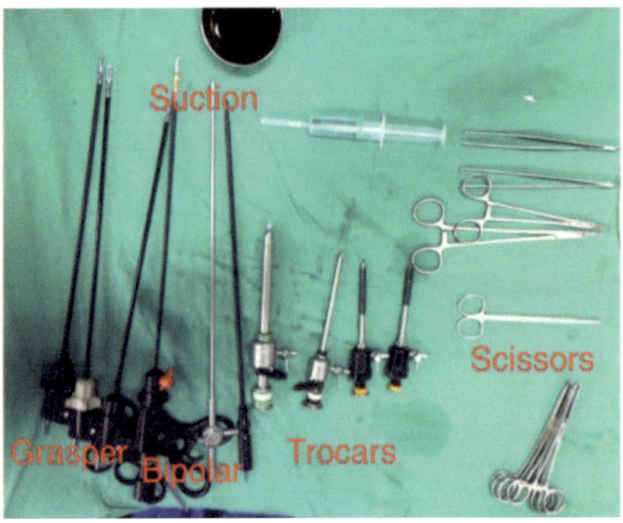

Figure 2. The laparoscopy instruments required are arranged in a sterile cart: grasper, bipolar, scissors, suction irrigation, trocars and cannula. One 10 mm and three 5 mm ports are necessary.

is on the right side of the patient. The second assistant does the uterine manipulation and he stands between the legs of the patient. A foam mattress is placed directly under the patient to prevent sliding during steep Trendelenburg. The table is kept in a low position to enable wrist movements for intracorporeal knotting. The monitor to directly face each surgeon at the angle of resting eye, i.e., 30°, to promote an ergonomic working environment. The surgeon, the target tissue and the monitor should be in straight line. The height of the table should be about the half of surgeons' height to enable wrist movements.

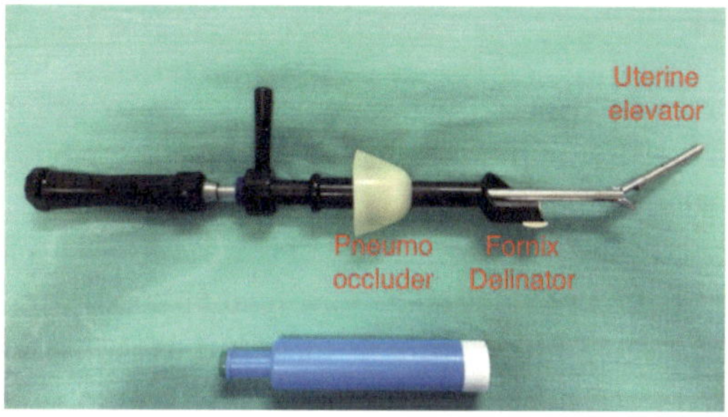

Figure 3. The uterine manipulator is used to antevert the uterus and delineate the fornixes for laparoscopic colpotomy. The pneumoperitoneum is maintained by the soft silastic parts of the instrument that prevent the air leak after colpotomy.

3.2. Vaginal manipulation

Uterine cannulation is performed with a specific instrument named The Clermont-Ferrand type Karl Storz Uterine Manipulator or RUMI - Uterine Manipulator (**Figure 3**).

First, a Sims speculum is placed into the vagina. Cervix is held with a tenaculum and the uterus is sounded. The cervix is dilated to Hegar number 9. RUMI tip used should be selected according to the patient after sounding the uterine cavity with a uterine sound. If the uterine cavity is 7, a 6-cm tip should be selected. The sizes available are 6, 8, or 10 cm. The distal end of the shaft may be dipped in the in lubricant prior to attaching the tip. This greatly facilitates the insertion into the uterine cavity. The pneumo-occluder is now slided over the tip and the shaft. Now the Koh cup (3, 3.5, and 4 cm in width) is attached. The Koh cup should be appropriately sized according to the cervix of the patient. This is important because a small ring will not mark the vaginal fornices exactly and only push up the cervix. The delineation of fornices is important because it serves as a landmark till the surgery is complete. A large ring will increase the risk of a ureteral injury. Insert the tip of the RUMI as far into the cervix as it will go. The correct placement is confirmed by palpation or direct visualization. Inflate the Uterine balloon with 5 cc of normal saline to manipulate the uterus and facilitate specimen removal through the vagina at the end of the case. The bladder is catheterized with Foleys catheter. The pneumo-occluder is now inflated with 60 to 100 cc of saline. RUMI II and RUMI arc are recent modifications that fascilate easy manipulation.

3.3. Establishing the pneumo-peritoneum

The stomach should be deflated by Ryle's tube insertion and aspiration. First step is to insert the Veress needle following the double click sound at subumbilical incision or the Palmer's point in the left upper quadrant, about 2 to 3 cm below the left costal margin, in the left mid-clavicular line [7]. Now, CO_2 insufflation is done to create pneumoperitoneum to achieve an intra-abdominal pressure of 12 to 14 mmHg [8, 9]. An easy way to confirm intraperitoneal entry is to look for the pressure reading on the insufflator. If the pressure reading is high the Veress needle is likely to be impinging on the omentum. A slight gentle movement will dislodge it. Alternatively bubble test can be done.

3.4. Positioning the trocar

Four trocars are positioned: one 10 mm umbilical trocar with a 30° optic and three 5 mm trocars, with one 2 cm medial to the right superior iliac crest, another 2 cm medial to the left anterior superior iliac crest, and a third in the midline, 8–10 cm below the umbilical port. These trocars are placed lateral to the rectus abdominis muscles, 2 cm above and 2 cm medial to the anterior superior iliac spine (**Figure 4**). The last 5 mm trocar can be substituted by a 10–15 mm trocar during surgery for the introduction of suture needles and for suturing of the vaginal vault. A complete survey of the abdomen to rule out any visceral injury at the time of entry is done. The lower quadrant trocar sleeves are placed under direct vision. In the case of very voluminous uteri, the trocars can be positioned more cephalad using the diamond baseball concept.

3.5. Visualization of pelvic organs

After inserting the ports the trocars are withdrawn and instruments are inserted. The patient is placed in 15° head low position to move the bowel loops away from pelvis. The small intestine loops are mobilized upwards to visualize the uterus, tubes, ovaries, round ligaments and infundibulopelvic ligaments. The surgeon uses a grasper and a bipolar and follows the manipulation angle of 60°. The Azimuth angle is maintained at 30°. Manipulation angle is the angle between the two operating instruments. Azimuth angle is the angle between the scope and the operating instrument. The first assistant holds the scope with the left hand and uses the Maryland grasper forceps in the right hand. If adhesions are seen they should be gently released. Releasing adhesions between sigmoid colon and utero-ovarian ligament permits the correct exposure of the infundibulopelvic ligament and posterior surface of the uterus. The sequence to be followed is look, hook, coagulate and cut. Thick tissue should be cauterized in small steps with coagulating cautery set at 35 W to prevent charring. The uterus is mobilized by the second assistant and is maintained cranially and anteriorly.

3.6. Coagulation and section of round ligament

The round ligament is secured with traction by the first assistant, making possible its exposure for the start of the surgery. The round ligament is coagulated at a distance of 2 to 3 cm from the lateral pelvic wall using a bipolar cautery (**Figure 5**). The coagulation of the round

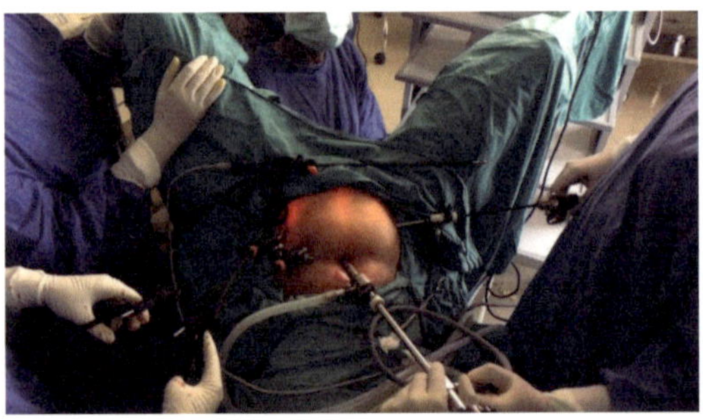

Figure 4. Laparoscopic port positions for total laparoscopic hysterectomy with ipsilateral ports. The infraumbilical port is the telescopic port. The right iliac fossa port is the traction port and the two left iliac fossa ports are the operating ports.

http://dx.doi.org/10.5772/intechopen.75652

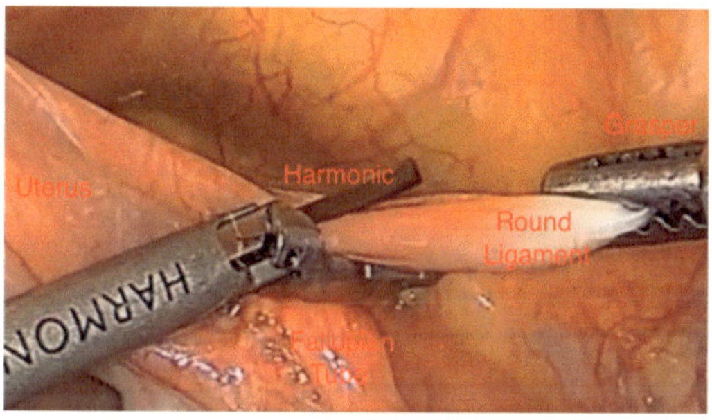

Figure 5. The round ligament is held 2–3 cm from the lateral pelvic wall. The ligament is coagulated with bipolar and cut with scissors.

ligament near the uterus is difficult as there is an artery to the round ligament which may bleed. This is followed by opening the anterior leaflet of the broad ligament to the vesico-uterine peritoneal reflection.

3.7. Coagulation and section of the infundibulo-pelvic ligament

The first assistant should secure the adnexa and apply traction in a direction opposite to the operating side (**Figure 6**). The coagulation and sectioning of the ligament should be progressive, plane to plane (peritoneum, followed by the vessels and connective tissue). The infundibulopelvic ligament or the tubo-ovarian ligament are now coagulated and with a bipolar grasper and scissors. The infundibulopelvic ligament should be coagulated close to the ovary (hug the ovary) as this helps to avoid injury to the vital structures in the pelvic sidewall. The tubo-ovarian ligament should also be coagulated close to the ovary to prevent injury to the uterine vessel during ovarian conservation. When you want to preserve the adnexa, the coagulation and section is performed proximal to the fallopian tubes and the utero-ovarian ligament. The posterior leaf of broad ligament is opened with incision extending till the internal os being careful not to injure the uterine artery and vein (**Figure 7**). The peritoneum is opened, coagulated and cut till the attachment of the utero-sacral ligaments. The capillaries in the posterior leaf of broad ligament and the parametrial veins that run between the ovary and round ligament should be taken care of.

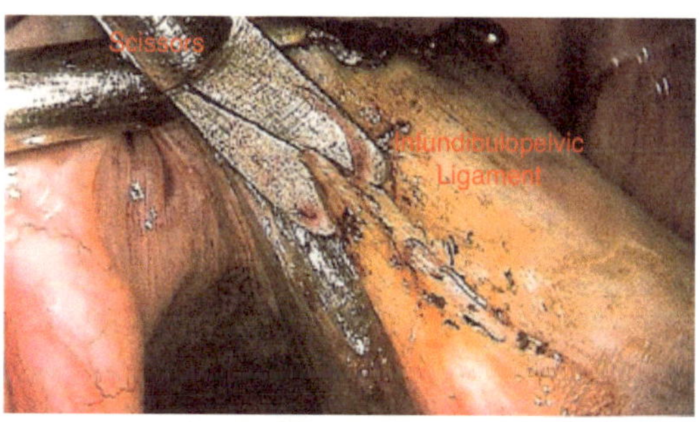

Figure 6. The infundibulopelvic ligament is identified by gentle traction. It is also coagulated with bipolar and cut with scissors.

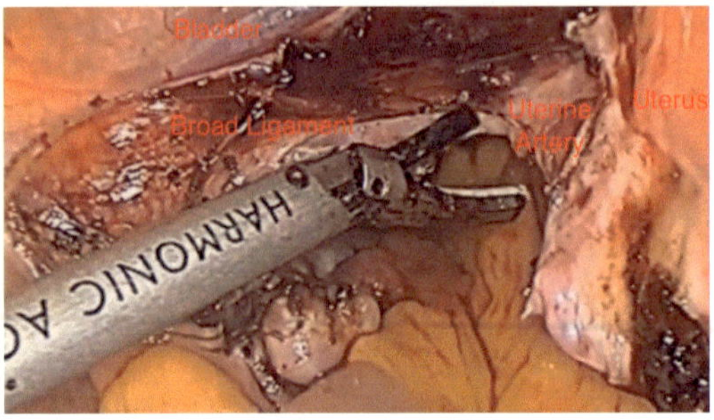

Figure 7. The peritoneum in the broad ligament is opened and uterine vessels are identified at the level of internal os.

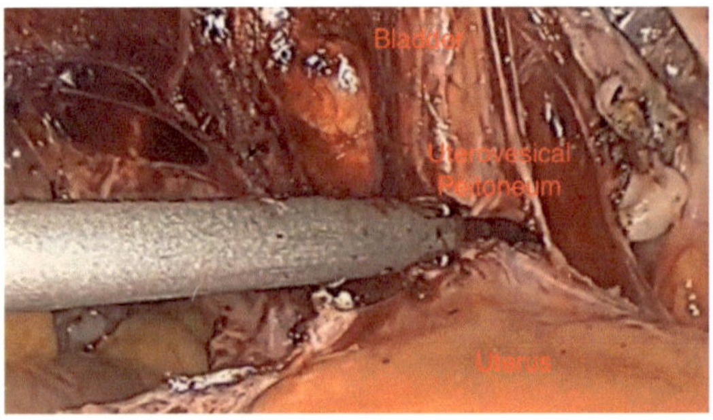

Figure 8. The loose vesicouterine fold of peritoneum is held with grasper and scissors used to dissect the bladder. The bladder is gently dissected downwards by laparoscopic pledgets or applying traction from the jaws of bipolar.

3.8. Mobilization of bladder

The assistant uses an atraumatic forceps to grasp the peritoneum and the bladder in the midline, applying vertical and cranial traction (**Figure 8**). The peritoneum and the adjacent connective tissue are coagulated and sectioned, thus accessing the vesico-vaginal plane and posteriorly to expose the bottom of vesico-uterine sac. The dissection continues in a caudal direction, initially in the midline and then laterally, performing the coagulation and section of the vesico-uterine ligaments thereby mobilizing the bladder off the lower uterine segment. The plane of loose areolar tissue should be identified and opened avoiding injury to the vessels. In women with previous cesarean delivery, there are adhesions between bladder and lower uterine surface and so dissection should be a little high as close to the uterus as possible to avoid bladder injury.it is important to identify and pick small bits of tissue close to the uterus and coagulate and cut them gradually moving down towards the cervix [10]. Alternatively a lateral approach of opening the broad ligament may be the preferred route [11, 12]. During laparoscopic hysterectomy, if the patient has significant adhesions from prior cesarean deliveries, a reverse inferior to superior vesico-uterine fold dissection can be used to dissect the bladder from the uterus [13]. This lateral dissection and accessing the bladder from below can be used as an alternative to the commonly practiced technique of mobilizing the bladder in a superior to inferior fashion at the time of laparoscopic hysterectomy. The anatomy of the space of Seth can be helpful in identifying the lateral structures of bladder. Space of Seth is bounded laterally by the tangential line joining the maximum bulging on the uterine body and cervix, medially the bladder comes in contact with the uterocervical surface thickening at the level of bladder pillars. Anteriorly there is the undersurface of bladder and anterior leaf of broad ligament, posteriorly there is the uterocervical surface [14].

A reevaluation of the route of dissection is advised if fat is encountered because the fat belongs to the bladder and this may indicate that the dissection is moving too close to the bladder. With this the ureter is kept out-of-the-way, since it is mobilized along with the peritoneum.

3.9. Secure uterine vessels

Desiccate the ascending uterine vessels with the bipolar grasper at the level of internal cervical os. The RUMI uterine can be pushed upwards to increase the distance between uterine artery and. The uterine vessels should coagulate till there is vaporization and bubble formation. The uterine vessels should be grasped perpendicularly to coagulate the 7 mm lumen efficiently. If the uterine are grasped obliquely the lumen to be coagulated becomes wider. Grasping the uterine artery perpendicularly is made easier by the new articulating instruments which can change direction and allow the uterine artery to be grasped and coagulated perpendicularly (**Figure 9**). After the coagulation and cutting of uterine arteries the vascular pedicles are deflected laterally and dissection is continued in the avascular plane over the cervix towards the delineated vaginal fornices (**Figure 10**). The ureters should be reconfirmed and the dissection continued close to the uterus [15].

3.10. Removal of uterus

While pushing cephalad with the uterine manipulator, vaginal fornices are identified. It is identified by indentation of the Rumi Koh colpotomizer or by palpation with a laparoscopic instrument. The Harmonic scalpel or laparoscopic monopolar hook is then used to cut circumferentially around the cup, thus uterus with cervix is separated from vaginal apex (**Figures 11** and **12**). In patients with limited vaginal access, the uterus can be morcellated using an electronic morcellator and specimen removed abdominally. It is important to keep the tip of the morcellator in clear view at all times.

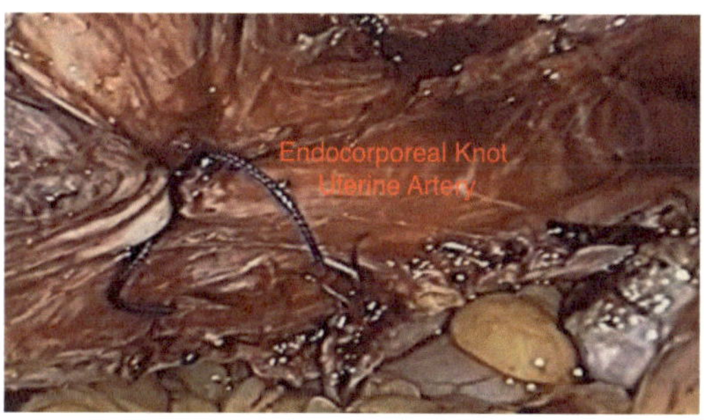

Figure 9. The uterine vessels are secured with endocorporeal knotting or harmonic.

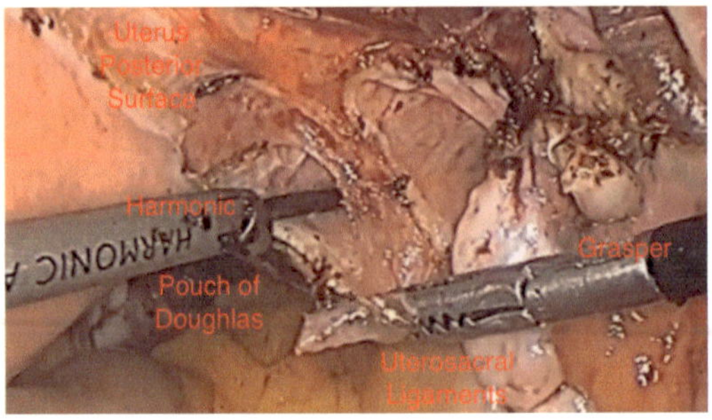

Figure 10. Uterosacral ligaments are identified and the peritoneal incision is extended to the pouch of douglas. The peritoneal incision is above the uterosacral ligaments.

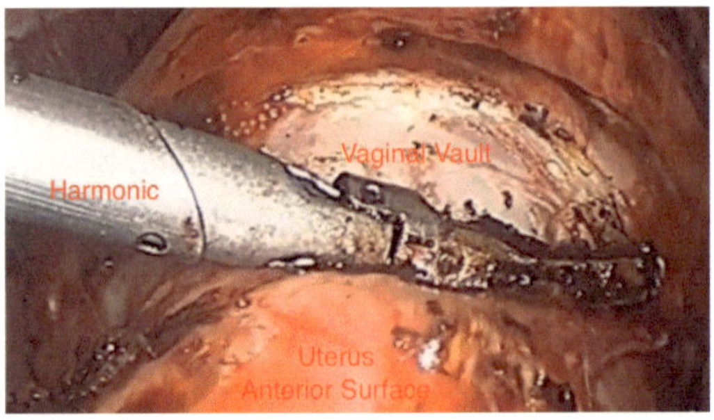

Figure 11. The vaginal vault is incised with a harmonic or laparoscopy monopolar hook after delineating the fornixes. The vaginal vault is incised above the attachment of uterosacral ligaments.

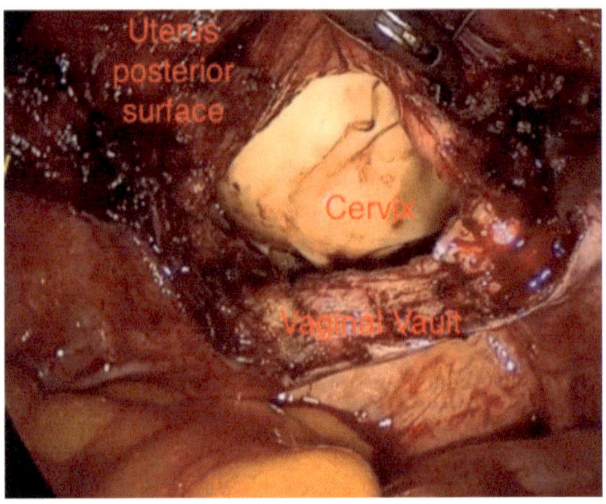

Figure 12. The posterior lip of cervix is seen after vaginal vault is incised. The pneumoperitoneum leakage is prevented by the RUMI manipulator in the vagina.

3.11. Vaginal cuff closure

Vaginal cuff should closed beginning at the margins of angle of the vaginal canal. The barb sutures are continued in running manner. The vaginal mucosa and the pubocervical and recto-vaginal fascia are included in the suture line. Each suture should be placed at 1 cm in distance from vaginal cuff margins. This is important and can be guessed as a comparison to the wide open jaw of grasper which is 2 cm wide. Distances can be easily underestimated because of the magnification of the laparoscope. Irrigation and suction is performed and hemostasis rechecked. The bidirectional barbed suture is available in which wound tension is evenly distributed across the length of the suture line rather than at the knotted end. No knots are required with bidirectional barbed suture. Since uterosacral ligament attachment to vagina is undisturbed in Total Laparoscopic hysterectomy the vaginal vault fixation is not required.

No routine cystoscopy is needed to ensure ureteral patency and bladder injury except in cases of dense bladder adhesions. However cystoscopy does not identify delayed thermal injury to ureters and bladder.

The pneumoperitoneum is deflated.

3.12. Port wound closure

The fascial defect of the 10 mm trocar in the midline is sutured and the skin is sutured with 3–0 monofilament absorbable suture.

Laparoscopic direct visualization fascial closure methods provide more accurate placement of sutures under direct vision.

Recommendations regarding port wound closure:

1. All ports greater than 10 mm either in midline or lateral should be closed at fascial level.
2. 5 mm ports if manipulated extensively or enlarged significantly during the procedure need to be closed
3. Port closure should include fascia and peritoneum.

The LigaSure Vessel Sealer, The EnSeal—Advanced Tissue Sealing Technology and the Ultracision ® harmonic scalpel are newer advances in laparoscopic surgery. Articulating vessel sealer helps to grasp and coagulate the vessel at right angle to the course of the vessel, thereby minimizing the diameter of vessel to be coagulated. Each surgeon should develop his own routine and use the available materials and technology to facilitate the surgical procedure.

4. Advantages of laparoscopic hysterectomy

1. Small surgical wound
2. Short hospital stay
3. Quick recovery
4. No abdominal wound
5. Decrease in intra op bleeding

6. Decrease in post op pain and infection
7. Low incidence of DVT.
8. Early return of bowel activity
9. Less risk of adhesion formation

5. Indications for conversion to open procedure

5.1. Planned conversion

1. Failure to progress
2. Dense or extensive lower abdominal or pelvic adhesions
3. Acute or chronic inflammatory changes causing increased vascularity resulting in tethering or tearing of tissues.
4. Difficulty to maintain pneumoperitoneum due to gas leaks in and around the ports.
5. Poor or inadequate exposure—obesity may preclude placement of ports
6. Altered or aberrant or unclear anatomy
7. Inexperience of the surgeon

5.2. Emergency conversion

1. Technical problem/instrument malfunction
2. Anesthesia related issues like—poorly tolerating pneumoperitoneum
3. Complex viscus injury

The surgeon should keep in mind the time of dissection and the progress made as well as the remaining tasks to be completed. Also the surgeon's threshold for conversion should be low while gaining experience.

6. Adhesion prevention during laparoscopic surgery

1. Minimize tissue damage
2. Perfect hemostasis
3. Minimize length of insufflation
4. Minimize intra-abdominal pressure
5. Adequate irrigation to avoid desiccation

6. Gentle tissue manipulation
7. Physical barriers like Seprafilm/Intercede

7. Post-operative pain management

There is a documented reduction in the narcotic requirement after laparoscopic Hysterectomy when compared to open procedure. It is also associated with earlier return of bowel function, earlier discharge, and improved pulmonary function.

Post op pain is due to irritation of somatic nerve fibers by overdistension of the diaphragm and carbon dioxide pneumoperitoneum related acidic intraperitoneal environment. Peritoneal ischemia, distension neurapraxia are other mechanisms that account for post op pain.

Method of reducing postoperative pain:

1. Infiltration of abdominal wall incision with local anesthetics
2. Intra peritoneal instillation of saline at the end of the procedure
3. Epidural analgesia
4. Complete removal of insufflated gas
5. Postoperative non-steroidal anti-inflammatory drugs

7.1. Prophylaxis against deep vein thrombosis

The addition of deep vein thrombosis prophylaxis should be at the discretion of the operating surgeon based upon the earlier recommendations and risk assessment of that particular patient.

7.2. Prevention of post-operative wound infection

1. Optimize the patient and iatrogenic risk factors.
2. Appropriate use of systemic perioperative antibiotics.
3. Adequate operative site preparation.
4. Avoid unnecessary trauma from hair removal techniques.
5. Avoid wiping off antiseptic after the skin preparation
6. Strict adherence to principles of sterility
7. Wide preparation of skin in case of conversion to laparotomy.
8. Adequate sized skin incisions will prevent ischemia and marginal wound necrosis.
9. Occlusive dressings to be released after 48 h because they might be conducive to bacterial overgrowth.

How to avoid Port site bleeding complications?

1. The trocar and the port should enter the abdomen at 90° to skin surface.
2. Dermal incision should be complete before using the trocar to penetrate the fascia.
3. Surgeon should be familiar with the mechanics of the given trocar.
4. Port placement should be made either in the midline or lateral to the edge of rectus sheath to avoid inferior epigastric artery.
5. Blunt tip ports are preferable to sharp tipped ones.

7.3. Post-operative advice

1. Advice to start on liquids after 6 h and to a regular light diet as tolerated on first day.
2. Bath after 48 h—for skin incision to re-epithelialize.
3. No restriction to walking from first post op day.
4. Resumption to preoperative activity by second week.
5. Regular exercise encouraged after 4 weeks.
6. Resumption of driving depends on mobility, reaction time, patient ability to respond to any road hazard. Usually resumes by 1–2 weeks.
7. Return to work by 2 weeks.
8. Continue Hematinics and Calcium supplements for 3 months.
9. Abstinence for 6 weeks.

7.4. How to avoid port site hernia

1. Minimum number of ports with smallest possible diameter.
2. Violent torqueing of port which can enlarge fascial defect.
3. Slow desufflation of abdomen while removing the ports—rapid removal of ports may draw bowel and omentum into port sites.
4. Before closure of ports shake the abdomen to dislodge the stuck bowel.
5. Closure of fascial defects before patient is extubated.

7.5. Port site seroma

It is a painless ballotable swelling at a healing port site. It usually occurs within 1–5 days post-operatively. There is no evidence of inflammation. It usually resolves spontaneously within days unless complicated by secondary bacterial infection.

7.6. Port site tumors

Port site tumor is common when an unexpected malignant specimen is retrieved through one of the ports. Serious complication has been noted in setting of ovarian cancer and to lesser extent in patients with endometrial cancer and rare in cervical cancer patients. The presence of 10–15 mm Hg pneumoperitoneum may facilitate the dispersion of liberated tumor cells throughout the abdomen and to port site during insufflation events. The employment of specimen bags is recommended to retrieve the specimen. Laparoscopic skill level of the surgeon also plays a critical factor.

8. Conclusion

Laparoscopy offers the advantage of clear magnified anatomy and pathology. The adhesions can be dissected carefully under vision. To minimize complications the basic principles that should be kept in mind can be summarized.

1. Proper patient selection
2. Adequate experience of the surgeon and assistants
3. Proper port placement
4. Avoid gas leaks
5. Sound surgical techniques
6. Adequate sized incisions
7. Thorough irrigation of port and abdomen before closure
8. Fascial and peritoneal wound closure for 10 mm or larger ports

Acknowledgements

Authors thank the nursing staff of Department of Obstetrics and Gynecology, Department of Radiology and Department of Anesthesiology, Saveetha Medical College, Chennai, for the care given to the women. We also thank the staff of Operation theaters and staff of blood bank. We thank the Biotechnical Department of Saveetha Medical College and hospital.

We also acknowledge the funds provided by Saveetha University, Chennai for the laparoscopy surgical care for women.

Conflict of interest

The authors declare that there is no conflict of interest.

Author details

Nidhi Sharma* and Vanusha Selvin

*Address all correspondence to: drbonuramkumar@yahoo.co.in

Saveetha Medical College, Saveetha University, Chennai, India

References

[1] Veres J. Neues instrument zur ausfuhrung von brust-oder bauchpunktionen und pneumothoraxbehandlung. Deutsche Medizinische Wochenschrift. 1938;**64**:1480-1481

[2] Reich H, DeCaprio J, McGlynn F. Laparoscopic hysterectomy. Journal of Gynecologic Surgery. 1989;**5**:213-216

[3] Reich H. Laparoscopic hysterectomy. Surgical Laparoscopy and Endoscopy. 1992;**2**:85-88

[4] Liu CY. Laparoscopic hysterectomy: A review of 72 cases. The Journal of Reproductive Medicine. 1992;**37**:351-354

[5] Liu CY. Laparoscopic hysterectomy. Report of 215 cases. Gynaecological Endoscopy. 1992;**1**:73-77

[6] Reich H, McGlynn F, Sekel L. Total laparoscopic hysterectomy. Gynaecological Endoscopy. 1993;**2**:59-63

[7] Palmer R. Instrumentation et technique de la coelioscopie gynecologique. Gynecologie Et Obstetrique (Paris). 1947;**46**:420-431. PMID 18917806

[8] Gould JC, Philip A. Principles and techniques of abdominal access and physiology of pneumoperitoneum. Scientific American Surgery. 2011;**8**:P1-P9

[9] Molloy D, Kaloo PD, Cooper M, et al. Laparoscopic entry: A literature review and analysis of techniques and complications of primary port entry. The Australian & New Zealand Journal of Obstetrics & Gynaecology. 2002;**42**:246-253

[10] Wang L, Merkur H, Hardas G, Soo S, Lujic S. Laparoscopic hysterectomy in the presence of previous caesarean section: A review of one hundred forty-one cases in the Sydney west advanced pelvic surgery unit. Journal of Minimally Invasive Gynecology. 2010;**17**(2):186-191. DOI: 10.1016/j.jmig.2009.11.007

[11] Sinha R, Sundaram M, Lakhotia S, Hedge A, Kadam P. Total laparoscopic hysterectomy in women with previous cesarean sections. Journal of Minimally Invasive Gynecology. 2010;**17**(4):513-517. DOI: 10.1016/j.jmig.2010.03.018. PMID: 20621012

[12] Celle C, Pomés C, Durruty G, Zamboni M, Cuello M. Total laparoscopic hysterectomy with previous cesarean section using a standardized technique: Experience of Pontificia Universidad Catolica de Chile. Gynecological Surgery. 2015;**12**(3):149-155

[13] Nezhat C, Grace LA, Razavi GM, Mihailide C, Bamford H. Reverse vesicouterine fold dissection for laparoscopic hysterectomy after prior cesarean deliveries. Obstetrics and Gynecology. 2016;**128**(3):629-633. DOI: 10.1097/AOG.0000000000001593. PMID: 27500328

[14] Sheth SS. Reverse vesicouterine fold dissection for laparoscopic hysterectomy after prior cesarean deliveries. Obstetrics & Gynecology. 2017;**129**(4):749-750. DOI: 10.1097/AOG.0000000000001954

[15] Manoucheri E, Cohen SL, Sandberg EM, Kibel AS, Einarsson J. Ureteral injury in laparoscopic gynecologic surgery. Reviews in Obstetrics and Gynaecology. 2012;**5**(2):106-111

Section 2

Tricks for a Better Laparoscopic Approach

Chapter 6

Handheld Devices for Laparoscopic Surgery

Francisco M. Sánchez-Margallo,
Juan A. Sánchez-Margallo and Amir Szold

Additional information is available at the end of the chapter

http://dx.doi.org/10.5772/intechopen.74117

Abstract

Despite the well-known benefits of minimally invasive surgery (MIS) to the patients, this surgical technique implies some technical challenges for surgeons. These technical limitations are increased with the introduction of laparoendoscopic single-site (LESS) surgery. In order to overcome some of these technical difficulties, new handheld devices have been developed, providing improved functionalities along with precision-driven and articulating instrument tips. In this chapter, we will review the current status of handheld devices for laparoscopy and LESS surgery. Devices that provide additional and innovative functionalities in comparison with conventional surgical instruments will be considered. Results will be based on studies published in the scientific literature and our experience. These surgical devices will be organized into two main groups, mechanical devices and robotic-driven devices. In general, these instruments intend to simulate the dexterity of movements of a human wrist. Mechanical devices are cheaper and easier to develop, so most of the available handheld instruments fall into this category. The majority of the robotic-driven devices are needle holders with an articulating tip, controlled by an interface implemented on the instrument handle. In general, these handheld devices claim to offer an enhancement of dexterity, precision, and ergonomics.

Keywords: handheld instruments, laparoscopic surgery, mechanical instruments, robotic instruments, robotic surgery

1. Introduction

The reduction of invasiveness in surgery has led to numerous benefits to the patients. However, minimally invasive surgery (MIS) implies some technical challenges for surgeons.

The less invasive the surgery, the more difficult it is to reach the surgical targets. MIS requires a close proximity of surgical instruments and the endoscopic camera, leading to a loss of instruments triangulation, restriction of maneuverability inside the abdominal cavity, and the adoption of uncomfortable body postures for long periods of time. These technical limitations are increased with the introduction of laparoendoscopic single-site (LESS) surgery, in which the freedom of movements of the surgical instruments is more restricted due to the single surgical access.

Conventional laparoscopic instruments have limited dexterity, making some surgical maneuvers challenging. The use of surgical ports creates a pivot point for the instruments in the body wall, which reduces the degrees of freedom (DoF) of the surgical instruments, from six (free motion) in conventional surgery to four in laparoscopic surgery, as illustrated in **Figure 1**. Besides, laparoscopic instruments suffer from ergonomically inadequate handle designs and inefficient transmission of force and tactile feedback from the handle to the instrument tip [1, 2].

All the aforementioned restrictions of surgeons' dexterity, in conjunction with the performance of repetitive tasks and the adoption of awkward and static postures during surgery, contribute to the onset of muscular fatigue and other musculoskeletal problems [2–4].

In order to overcome some of these technical limitations, new handheld devices have been developed for laparoscopic surgery and LESS surgery. These novel devices provide precision-driven and articulating instrument tips in combination with improved functionalities. They

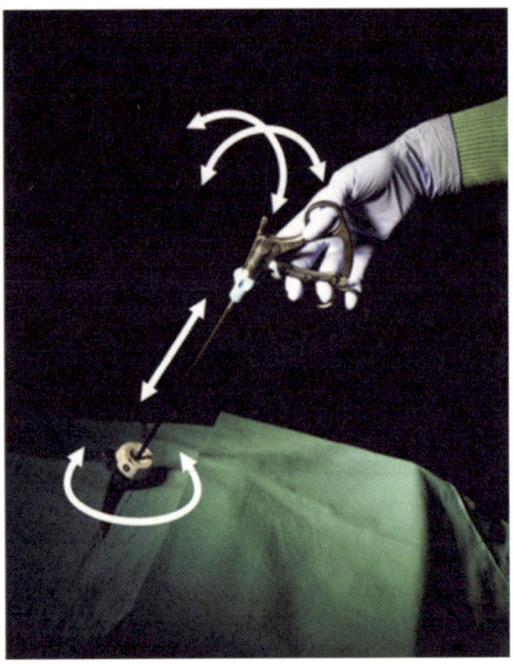

Figure 1. Illustration of the four degrees of freedom when using laparoscopic instruments.

aim at enhancing surgical dexterity, increasing instrument triangulation, and thus, improving the performance of certain surgical maneuvers. This optimization and improvement of the surgical instruments arise as a response to the complex surgical procedures that are now possible through laparoscopic and single-site surgical approaches.

Although there are other innovative alternatives such as the robotic surgical platforms (e.g., the da Vinci® Surgical System), these systems are associated with substantial financial and maintenance costs [5]. Therefore, a great interest in both academic and commercial institutions has arisen in creating devices that can provide some of the advantages of these robotic surgical platforms, but at a lower cost, filling the space between conventional surgical instruments and surgical robotics. In this context, innovative handheld laparoscopic devices have emerged. These devices are mainly divided into two categories: handheld mechanical instruments and handheld robotic devices. Systems falling into each category will be described in the following sections. This article will give an overview of the state-of-the-art in handheld instruments for laparoscopic surgery and LESS surgery. Only surgical instruments that provide a clear evidence of significant development and additional features when compared to conventional MIS instruments will be addressed.

2. Handheld mechanical instruments

Control interfaces for mechanical surgical instruments with articulating end effectors can be mainly classified as handle control, thumb control, and mixed control [5, 6]. For the handle control interface, the instrument handle is articulated relative to the instrument shaft, which makes the instrument tip steer. In the thumb control method, the movements of the instrument tip are controlled by a thumb interface generally paced on the instrument handle. The mixed control interface consists of a combination of the handle and the thumb control, including knobs and levers to control the instrument tip [6].

2.1. Laparoscopic surgery

Most of the handheld devices have been developed for their use during laparoscopic surgery. However, as it will be shown below in this section, some of them have been also tested in LESS surgery.

2.1.1. Radius r2 DRIVE (Tuebingen Scientific Medical GmbH, Tübingen, Germany)

The previous version of the r2 DRIVE instrument was the Radius Surgical System [7], which was a reusable needle holder with a shaft diameter of 10 mm but slightly shorter than conventional laparoscopic instruments with 50 cm in length. The r2 DRIVE instruments provide a 90-degree deflectable and infinite rotatable tip. They have a handle with a lever that deflects unidirectionally with respect to the shaft, in order to control the flexion of the instrument tip and a knob for the tip rotation, providing a total of seven DoF. One of the main advantages of the Radius Surgical System is that it can be sterilized and disassembled for cleaning. Improvements of this device over conventional laparoscopic instruments have been shown regarding safety and ergonomics [7]. However, it seems that the instrument is not very intuitive, and it requires a significant amount of practice to learn how to be used [8]. This instrument has already been tested in LESS surgery for suturing and ligation during a common bile duct exploration with C-tube drainage for choledocholithiasis [9] and for suturing during a laparoscopic transabdominal preperitoneal hernioplasty [10].

The new version, the r2 DRIVE, has a handle design similar to the Radius Surgical System and with the same mechanism of actuation but with a shaft diameter of 5 mm and the possibility of bipolar electrocautery [11]. A multifinger trigger on the handle operates the opening and closing actions of the jaws. The operating mechanism of this instrument is based on gears to deflect and rotate the end effector (**Figure 2**). This device enables to use different type of instruments, including scissors, dissectors and needle holder. However, the r2 DRIVE version is not sterilizable and has only one use.

There are no studies proving the feasibility of the r2 DRIVE instruments in an actual surgical setting. The technical utility and training effect of these instruments were evaluated during laparoscopic gastro-jejunal anastomoses in an ex vivo porcine model performed by a group of three experienced surgeons and four novices [12]. During this surgical task, execution time and anastomotic quality were analyzed. Results showed that after a limited number of cases, a stable mean anastomotic times and a fast learning curve were obtained.

2.1.2. FlexDex® (FlexDex Inc., Brighton, MI, USA)

The FlexDex® surgical instrument precisely translates the surgeon's hand, wrist, and arm movements from outside the patient into the respective movements of the end effector inside the patient's body in an intuitive manner. This instrument is based on a simple and mechanical

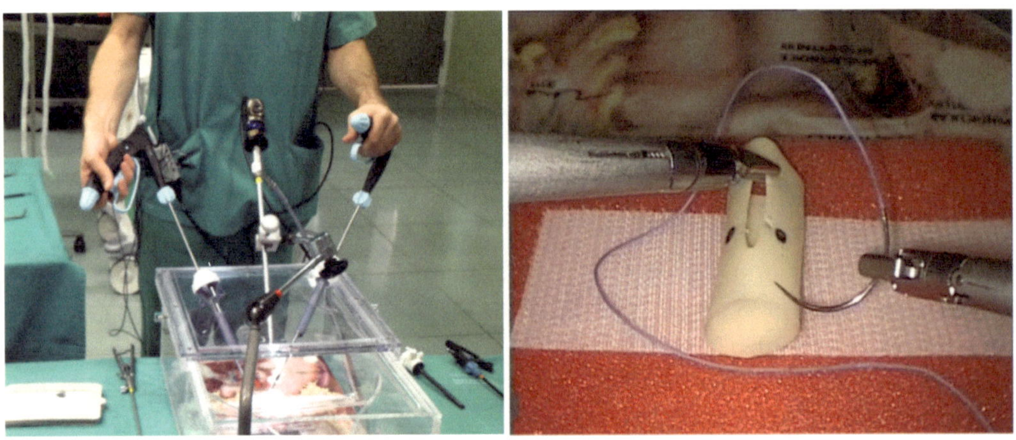

Figure 2. Use of the r2 DRIVE instruments on a box trainer (left). Performance of a laparoscopic suturing task (right).

design with no electrical components. This has a tool frame attached to the user's forearm which acts as an interface to transmit the movements from the forearm, wrist, and hand to the instrument tip. This interface mechanism provides a direct transmission of the three translations and roll rotation of the surgeon's forearm to the tool shaft and the end effector. In addition, the two wrist rotations of the surgeon's hand are transferred to the end-effector via transmission strips, pulleys, and cables [13]. The opening and closing movements of the instrument tip are controlled by a thumb lever on the instrument handle. Consequently, it allows FlexDex® to provide similar degrees of freedom to the surgeon's wrist.

As regards limitations of this instrument, the use of the forearm-brace may be time consuming to wear for surgery and wear off when the surgeon wants to change the surgical instrument. Besides, the tool frame keeps the instrument shaft parallel to the forearm, which may conflict with other instruments, reducing the location options of the instruments' entry ports into the patient's abdominal cavity [5, 14].

Criss et al. presented the initial use of the FlexDex® needle holder in a case of a reoperative laparoscopic Nissen fundoplication in a 2-year-old male patient [14]. They reported that the instrument provides articulated and intuitive control and successfully enables suturing and knot tying in limited spaces. However, additional studies are needed in order to analyze the reliability and learning curve of this instrument. This device is a commercial product, but it is currently only sold in the territory of the United States.

2.2. LESS surgery

Conflict of instruments, lack of triangulation, and difficult retraction are some of the biggest factors that limit the use of current surgical instruments during LESS surgery [15, 16]. Most of the surgical instruments for laparoscopic surgery are not completely suitable for LESS surgery, hampering its use during surgery. Articulating instruments have been designed to deal with some of these challenges inherent in LESS surgeries, improving the triangulation of the instruments inside the patient. In this section, we will review some of the most popular mechanical handheld instruments for LESS surgery. We have kept outside of this article the pre-bent shape instruments. These instruments do not allow to change their shape during its use in surgery, and they do not provide other additional functionalities.

2.2.1. *RealHand® (Novare Surgical System, Cupertino, CA, USA)*

These handheld instruments have 5 mm of shaft diameter with a pistol handle with rings and wrist control. The end effector is cable-driven with reverse kinematic mapping, which enables 360 degrees of articulation and a total of seven degrees of freedom (DoF). The instruments comprise a cautery, a grasper, a dissector, and a ThermaSeal (seals and separates tissue). The instrument design has a locking mechanism that allows for its use as a regular straight instrument or with multiple DoF [15].

The use of these instruments was evaluated in 10 patients who underwent a laparoscopic-assisted vaginal hysterectomy for the treatment of stage I uterine cancer [17]. Results showed no intraoperative or postoperative complications and normal levels of blood loss. Surgeons indicated that the instrument articulation appears to allow for more accurate targeting of nodes. Another study analyzed the joint forces of this flexible instrument and compared them with the actual force required to secure surgical ties for the ureter, renal artery, and renal vein [18]. They concluded that the joint forces developed by articulating instruments are not sufficient to meet the usual operative needs.

2.2.2. SILS® Hand (Medtronic, Minneapolis, MN, USA)

The SILS® Hand instruments offer different articulated surgical devices specially designed for LESS surgery in the form of hook, clinch, shears, and dissectors. These instruments have a pistol handle with rings and an articulation lock lever. They provide, by means of a reverse kinematic mapping, infinite positions of dynamic articulation of the tip. The instrument shaft can be articulated up to 80 degrees, and the tip has 360 degrees of rotation [16]. These articulated instruments have been widely used in LESS surgery for procedures such as colectomy [19], myomectomy [15], and partial nephrectomy [20], among others.

2.2.3. Radius r2 CURVE (Tuebingen Scientific Medical GmbH, Tübingen, Germany)

These instruments are 10-mm disposable instruments, which have a curved rotatable shaft, expressly designed for LESS surgery. As the r2 DRIVE version, these instruments have the same handle design and actuation mechanism, providing a 90-degree deflectable and infinite rotatable tip [21]. The flexion of the instrument tip is performed by deflecting the instrument handle and its rotation by using the knob on the handle. The specific shaft/tip design helps to avoid conflicts between instruments and the laparoscope during surgery, avoiding to occlude the view of the surgical field.

The feasibility of using this type of instruments was tested during LESS nephrectomy in a porcine model [12]. All LESS nephrectomies performed in a total of three pigs using the r2 CURVE instruments were successful without major complications. No conflicts between the handles of the two instruments used were reported. Besides, in order to avoid potential clashes between the camera and the instrument handles, an extra-long laparoscope was used during surgery.

2.2.4. Autonomy Laparo-Angle® (Cambridge Endoscopic Devices, Framingham, MA, USA)

This articulating instrument has a sword-like ergonomic handle shape, with reverse kinematic mapping between the instrument handle and the end effector, a 5-mm instrument shaft, and a flexible instrument tip. The axial rotation of the instrument tip is controlled by a knob mechanism implemented on the handle. This instrument has a locking system of the angle of flexion integrated in the handle. This may reduce the surgeons' muscle fatigue when they have to keep the instrument flexed. The distal instrument tip bends at any direction and turns 360 degrees at any angle, allowing for seven DoF. Unlike other flexible instruments for LESS surgery, this instrument enables to rotate, open and close the distal jaws after locking the instrument [15].

A retrospective study presented by Kim et al. [22] analyzed the medical records of 59 patients who underwent a myomectomy through a LESS approach and 59 patients using a traditional multiport approach. For the LESS myomectomy, surgeons used the Autonomy Laparo-Angle® for intracorporeal suturing, in combination with a handmade surgical port made out of a surgical glove and commercial trocars. In order to consider the surgeon's learning curve, records for the LESS approach were collected after 100 surgeries performed. Both approaches obtained similar results as far as operative time, estimated blood loss, postoperative hemoglobin drop, postoperative hospital stay, and postoperative pain scores are concerned.

3. Robotic-driven devices

Novel motor-driven, handheld devices that offer improved handle designs, functionalities, and precision-driven articulating end effectors have recently been introduced on to the medical market. The interface to control the instrument tip and other functionalities is usually located on the instrument handle. Some of these devices also allow surgeons to adjust the speed of the instrument movements according to their preference.

3.1. Laparoscopic surgery

3.1.1. Robot DEX™ (Dextérité surgical, Annecy, France)

This robotic instrument is a motor-driven laparoscopic needle holder, available on the market with a 10-mm instrument shaft. This consists of a console, a wired ergonomic handle, and a flexible tip with unlimited rotation. The flexion and rotation of the instrument tip are controlled by an interface on the handle. The instrument handle is a grip-type handle, which is connected by a mechanical joint to the instrument shaft. This grants surgeons greater freedom of movements, since the handle works independently from the shaft, which helps avoid forced movements of the wrist. This surgical tool provides a total of seven DoFs [23].

This device has been tested during a set of three different intracorporeal suturing tasks on a box trainer [23]. Precision using the surgical needle, quality of the intracorporeal suturing performance, execution time, and leakage pressure for the urethrovesical anastomosis, as well as the ergonomics of the surgeon's hand posture, were analyzed and compared with the use of a conventional laparoscopic needle holder. Results showed that, although both instruments offer similar technical performance, the robotic-driven instrument results in better ergonomics for the surgeon's hand posture during intracorporeal suturing. Besides, we recently conducted a study in which five experienced laparoscopic surgeons performed an urethrovesical anastomosis in a porcine model using the DEX™ system (unpublished study) (**Figure 3**). Participants used both a conventional axial-handled laparoscopic needle holder and the robotic instrument. Execution time, surgeon's posture, and pressure exerted by the surgeon's hand were assessed. Results revealed that the DEX™ system led to better ergonomics for the surgeon's hand, without differences in muscle fatigue between instruments. The robotic device required applying less pressure on the handle by the surgeons during surgery.

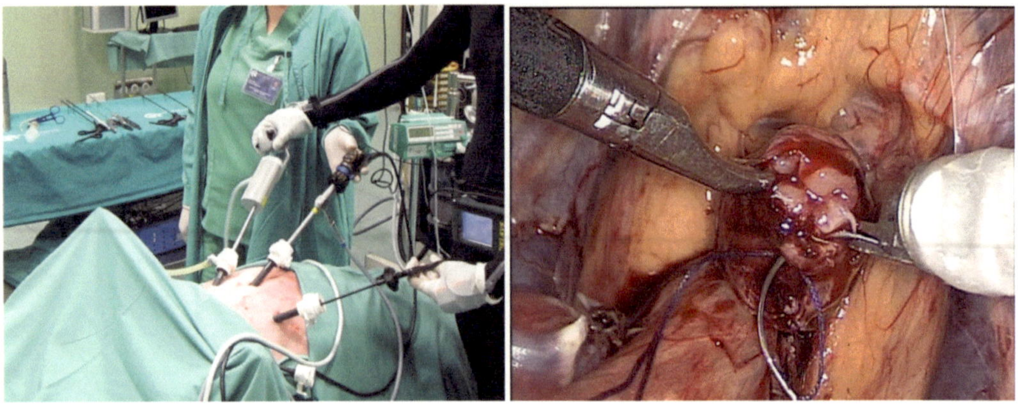

Figure 3. Use of the Robot DEX® robotic needle holder during an urethrovesical anastomosis in a porcine model.

3.1.2. JAiMY (Endocontrol, Grenoble, France)

This device is a 5-mm robotized needle holder available on the market with two additional intracorporeal DoF: yaw and roll. This instrument has a joystick placed on the handle to control the end effector, which can be used by right-handed and left-handed surgeons. The instrument tip can be bent up to 80 degrees and rotated, including speed control, by means of the joystick on the instrument handle.

Bensignor et al. [24] evaluated the effect of this instrument on the surgeon's skills and ergonomics during the performance of three basic suturing tasks on simulator. Performance outcomes, skills outcomes, and ergonomics were assessed. Performance outcomes were measured using a quantitative and qualitative score, and skills outcomes were measured by the number of movements and the path length traveled by the instrument. The RULA method was used for the surgeon's postural analysis [2, 25]. Muscular activity was assessed by means of electromyography of six muscular groups. The performance score was higher for the conventional instrument during the peg transfer task and for the JAiMY® instrument during the frontal suture task. Results showed an improved posture using the robotic instrument, but the muscular workload was lower for the conventional needle holder regarding the flexor carpi ulnaris and the triceps. The flexor carpi ulnaris is used for the opening and the closing of the jaws through the instrument trigger. The total path traveled by the instrument during the three tasks was shorter with the robotic device. Another study showed that an end effector with additional degrees of freedom combined with improved handle design increases ergonomics during laparoscopy and facilitates the performance of complex gestures [26].

3.1.3. Kymerax™ (Terumo Europe NV, Leuven, Belgium)

The Kymerax™ system is a handheld laparoscopic instrument with articulating and interchangeable instruments (scissors, dissector, needle holder, and L-hook) with a shaft diameter

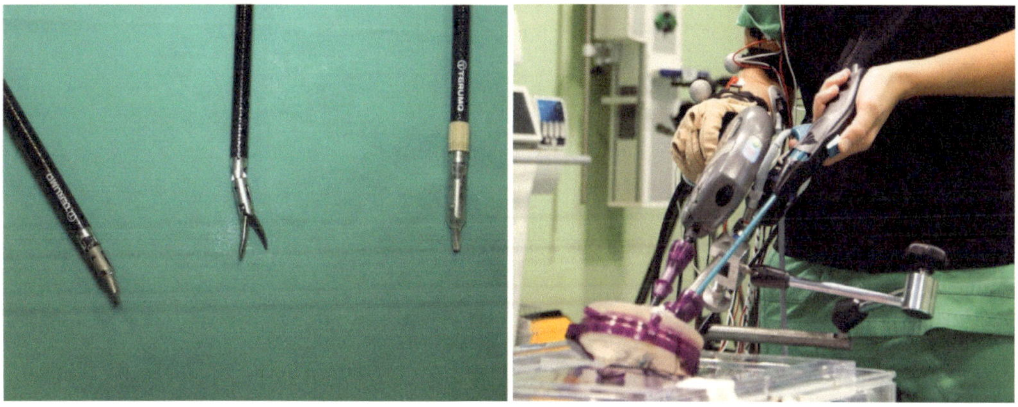

Figure 4. Interchangeable instruments (needle holder, dissector, and scissors) of the Kymerax® system. Use of the robotic device during LESS training tasks on a box trainer.

of 8.8 mm, which are driven by robotic technology (**Figure 4**). Surgeons control the movements of the instrument tip through the joystick interface implemented on the handle.

The efficacy of this robotic instrument has been tested with the European training in basic laparoscopic urologic skills (E-BLUS) and anastomosis tasks on a box trainer [27, 28]. During these tasks, surgeons used both 2D and 3D visualization systems. Results of this study showed that the combination of this device with 3D visualizing system led to a more successful completion of E-BLUS tasks for the novice surgeons and an increase of performance and quality of tasks during the anastomosis. Although surgeons rated the weight of this instrument as appropriate [27], analysis of the muscular intervention revealed a higher activity of the biceps muscle using the robotic device in comparison to a conventional needle holder, which may be associated with the increase of weight of this instrument [29].

This robotic device has been also used during clinical cases in laparoscopy. The first clinical use of this device in gynecological laparoscopy for malignant disease was described by Iacoponi et al. [30]. They presented the use of the Kymerax® instrument during laparoscopic hysterectomy for uterine sarcoma. They reported an operative time of 80 min, which is comparable to the time required for conventional laparoscopy, but less than the time required for robotic surgery [30, 31]. This robotic device has also been successfully used in LESS urological surgery [29, 32]. These studies will be discussed in the next section.

3.2. LESS surgery

The number of handheld robotic devices, excluding robotic platforms, specifically designed or employed in LESS surgery is scarce. The only robotic device commercially available that has been used during LESS urological and digestive procedures is the Kymerax™ system.

Device	Type	Instrument	Handle	DoF	Diameter (mm)	Clinical setting	Tasks/ procedures	References
Autonomy Laparo-Angle® (Cambridge Endoscopic Devices, Framingham, MA, USA)	Mechanical	Needle holder	Pistol	7	5	OR	LESS myomectomy	[22]
FlexDex® (FlexDex Inc., Brighton, MI, USA)	Mechanical	Needle holder	Forearm mounted	6	–	OR	Laparoscopy Nissen fundoplication	[14]
Jaimy® (Endocontrol, Grenoble, France)	Robot-driven	Needle holder	Pistol	6	5	Box trainer	Peg transfer Suturing tasks	[24]
Kymerax® (Terumo Europe NV, Leuven, Belgium)	Robot-driven	Scissors Dissector Needle holder L-hook	Pistol	5	8.8	Box trainer Ex vivo porcine model OR	European training in basic laparoscopic urological skills (E-BLUS) Anastomosis tasks Laparoscopic hysterectomy LESS partial nephrectomy LESS sigmoidectomy LESS radical prostatectomy	[27–30, 32]
r2 CURVE (Tuebingen Scientific Medical GmbH, Tübingen, Germany)	Mechanical	Scissors Dissector Needle holder	Pistol with a lever mechanism	7	5	Animal model	LESS nephrectomy	[12]
r2 DRIVE (Tuebingen Scientific Medical GmbH, Tübingen, Germany)	Mechanical	Scissors Dissector Needle holder	Pistol with a lever mechanism	7	5	Box trainer Ex vivo porcine model	Cutting and suturing tasks Gastro-jejunal anastomoses	[12]
RealHand® (Novare Surgical system, Cupertino, CA, USA)	Mechanical	Cautery Grasper Dissector ThermaSeal	Handle with rings	7	5	OR	Laparoscopic-assisted vaginal hysterectomy	[18]
Robot DEX® (Dextérité Surgical, Annecy, France)	Robot-driven	Needle holder	Grip-type	7	10	Box trainer	Precision task Suture on porcine stomach Urethrovesical anastomosis	[23]
SILS® Hand (Medtronic, Minneapolis, MN, USA)	Mechanical	Dissector Sears Clinch Hook	Handle with rings	7	5	OR	Colectomy Myomectomy Partial nephrectomy	[15, 19, 20]

Table 1. Summary of the handheld surgical instruments for laparoscopic and LESS surgery.

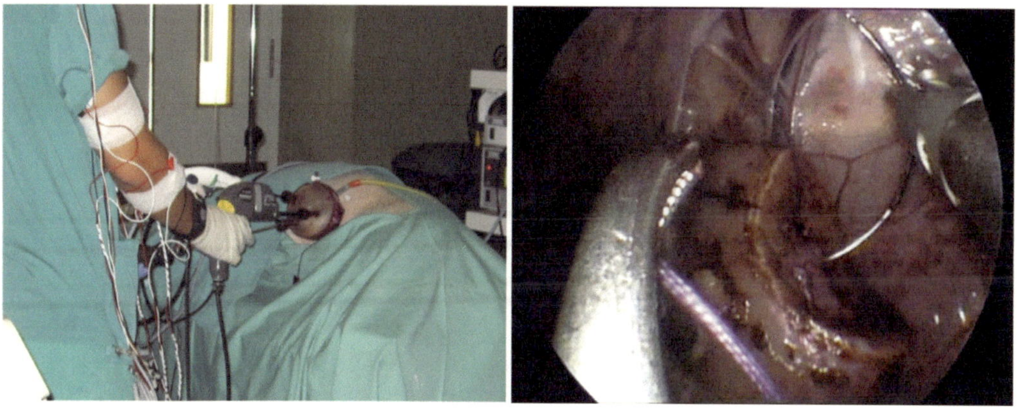

Figure 5. Partial nephrectomy in a porcine model using the Kymerax™ device.

Apart from the previous studies in laparoscopic surgery, the feasibility of this handheld robotic device has been also proved in LESS surgery [29]. The surgeon's performance and ergonomics using this robotic system during intracorporeal suturing tasks and digestive and urological procedures using a LESS approach were assessed. Surgeons performed an urethrovesical anastomoses on a simulator using an ex vivo porcine bladder, and a partial nephrectomy and a sigmoidectomy, in an in vivo experimental porcine model (**Figure 5**). Execution times, leakage pressure for the anastomosis, surgical complications, and surgeons' muscle intervention were measured and compared with the use of conventional laparoscopic instruments. Results showed similar outcomes in surgical performance and ergonomics using conventional laparoscopic instruments and the handheld robotic device. Muscle activity of the biceps was significantly higher using the robotic instrument during both surgical procedures. This may be due to the increased weight of the robotic device. Pérez et al. also presented a video article describing a laparoendoscopic hybrid single-site radical prostatectomy assisted by the Kymerax™ system [32]. The reported negative surgical margins and 0.03 ng/mL of PSA for the first month postoperative.

Table 1 shows a summary of the handheld devices analyzed in this chapter, including some of their main features and their relevant associated studies.

4. Other handheld devices

In this section, we will review the handheld devices for laparoscopic surgery that are still in a prototype phase or there is a lack of studies that demonstrate their feasibility in surgery.

4.1. Intuitool (University of Nebraska, Lincoln, NE, USA)

This laparoscopic instrument is a prototype with an ergonomically designed handle. This device has a thumb trackball placed on the instrument handle to control the end effector, which enables up to 60 degrees of articulation. The opening and closing actions of the jaws are controlled by a trigger implemented on the handle.

Trejo et al. [33] conducted a user study to evaluate this prototype. They found that 58% of the respondents believed the Intuitool would relieve hand/wrist pain due to inappropriate postures, and 53% believed the tool would reduce hand/wrist stiffness. In another study, Rousek et al. [34] analyzed different configurations in order to implement an electrosurgical hand control on the instrument handle. They sought preventing from causing poor ergonomic posture and physical discomfort due to the electrosurgical equipment operated by means of one or more foot pedals [34].

4.2. Hand-Held Robotic Device for Laparoscopy (University of Minho, Braga, Portugal; Polytechnic Institute of Cavado and Ave, Barcelos, Portugal)

This is a robotic device that includes disposable instruments with a bipolar system. The device weighs 730 g, has two speed modes (normal and fast speed), and can operate with a battery [35]. The rotation of the instrument tip is controlled by a joystick placed on the left side of the instrument handle. Surgeons interact with this joystick using their thumb. This device was designed only for right-handed surgeons. Besides, this only provides one additional DoF and the instrument tip cannot be flexed.

This robotic instrument in combination with 3D laparoscopic vision was tested by 26 surgeons during the performance of three basic laparoscopic tasks in a box trainer such as peg transfer, wire chaser, and knot tying [35]. Results showed that this device helps novice surgeons in reducing the time to complete the laparoscopic knot tying task. Novice surgeons stated that the combination with three-dimensional vision made their laparoscopic performance easier.

4.3. The Human Extensions Tool (Human Extensions, Netanya, Israel)

This instrument consists of a handheld electromechanical system that can support several end effectors with articulating tip. The system is cordless, lightweight, does not require any set up time, and can be easily moved between laparoscopic trocars and perform complex movements in a wide variety of complex minimally invasive operations. The instrument is composed of a sophisticated user interface that enables unrestricted hand movements. The surgeon operates the tools by using natural hand motions as if he/she was performing direct manual surgery on the patient.

4.4. OptiGrip™ (Endoscopic Force-reflecting Instruments B.V., Malden, The Netherlands)

This is the first grasper with haptic feedback for laparoscopic surgery. The main aim of this technology is to overcome the lack of tissue feedback in laparoscopic surgery when compared to traditional open surgery. This instrument translates the viscoelastic tissue feeling from the instrument tip to the trigger of the handle, resulting in more control and safer tissue manipulation. The instrument handle is available in small and large sizes to optimally fit in hands with different anthropomorphic features. This device can be set to different sensitivity levels for

http://dx.doi.org/10.5772/intechopen.74117

specific tissue types and with different visco-elastic properties. A study showed that enhanced haptic feedback may reduce the interaction force between instrument and tissues during surgery. Therefore, this may lead to less tissue damage, fewer complications, shorter operation times, and improved ergonomics [36].

4.5. Articulated Universal Joint for Minimally Invasive Surgery (Imperial College London, London, UK)

This is an articulated robotic device based on universal joints with embedded micromotors for minimally invasive surgery. This device provides a flexible tip with seven DoF, and it has two internal channels of 3 mm of diameter, one for an on-board camera for visualization and the other for passing interventional instruments. The articulated design allows the robot to explore the large areas of the peritoneal cavity. The handle can be decoupled from the articulated shaft, so it can be used to manipulate other instruments when it is necessary. The surgeon interacts with the instrument by means of a handle featuring a thumb-stick with an embedded push switch [37].

This handheld device has been used during a natural orifice transluminal endoscopic surgery (NOTES) tubular ligation procedure on an ex vivo model [37]. Surgeons reported some complications passing an endoscopic clip through the instrument channel due to the sharp edges at the tip. They solved the problem replacing the internal sheath of the instrument.

4.6. Maestro (Vanderbilt University, Nashville, TN, USA)

This prototype for laparoscopic surgery has been developed at the Vanderbilt University, and one of its main features is that it allows both parallel and reverse kinematic mappings between the instrument handle and the tip [5]. The end effector of the instrument is driven by tendons, and the open and close actions of the jaws are controlled by squeezing the two handle arms toward one another. This device also includes a locking mechanism for suturing tasks.

5. Discussion

Despite the numerous advantages associated with minimally invasive surgery (MIS), there are some technical limitations during its practice. These constraints are, in some cases, augmented by the use of novel surgical techniques such as LESS surgery. In this sense, the application of technology in surgery can make a huge contribution in order to address some of these limitations, such as the development of novel handheld devices for MIS with articulating end effectors. Handheld steerable instruments are preferred by surgeons due to their maneuverability during surgical procedures [6]. In general, the handheld surgical instruments presented in this chapter provide cost-effective methods of articulation, increasing the surgeon's intra-abdominal DoF. Most of these devices are articulated manual laparoscopic instruments which provide wrist-like dexterity to surgeons. These new mechanical and robotized handheld devices seem to be the future of MIS as they can increase both ergonomics and dexterity, resulting in an improvement of the quality of the surgical procedure.

Previous research has shown that ergonomics of the instrument handle influences on the task performance achieved with articulating laparoscopic instruments [38]. In this sense, Zahrahee et al. suggested that a finger-operated joystick control handle is easier to use and leads to a less fatigue than an articulating handle such as the RealHand® [39]. Besides, Fan et al. found no differences between thumb control and wrist control in terms of task performance [40]. We consider that it is fundamental to analyze the effect of a novel surgical instrument on the surgeon's ergonomics and performance. In this regard, several studies have been published for some of the handheld instruments that have been recently introduced in the market [23, 24, 29]. However, we consider that these studies should be done at an early stage prior to the final production and market launch.

Regarding the kinematic mapping of the mechanical instruments, the best direction of kinematic mapping is currently under discussion. For surgical approaches such as LESS, where instrument shafts must be near, parallel, and close to one another, a parallel mapping can potentially reduce the risk of the conflicts between instruments [5].

Both the instrument joints and the user interface for controlling the end effector are crucial aspects for the application of handheld articulating instruments in MIS. Flexible instruments with one or two steering segments at the tip allow for six DoF in the surgical scenario. Multiple steering segments can shape curved pathways inside the patient's abdominal wall. However, the development of multisegmented maneuverable instruments is still at an early stage [6]. Regarding the user interface, some instruments rotate the shaft itself, while others rotate the end effector using internal mechanisms controlled by a thumb knob or a wheel. In the case of the robotic devices, they operate the rotation of the instrument tip by means of a set of controls implemented on the handle.

Concerning the mechanical handheld instruments, not all of them incorporate a locking mechanism, which can be an inconvenient for some surgical tasks such as suturing. One positive aspect of using robotic-driven instruments is that surgeons can keep the instrument jaws closed without high physical demand. This action is assisted by the electromechanic technology of these devices.

The articulating power of articulating instruments is usually considered as suboptimal [18, 41]. Some of these instruments have some limitations to maintain the configuration of the instrument joints to grasp, carry, and transmit force [18]. Therefore, many surgeons prefer to use an articulating laparoscopic instrument in one hand and a conventional laparoscopic instrument in the other hand. One of the main reasons for this shortcoming is that articulating mechanisms are similar to those used for flexible endoscopes, so they are based on bendable plastics, steered by wires [18]. Some alternatives have been developed to cope with this problem such as solid joint frameworks, motor driven technologies, or pre-bent instruments. The main limitation of the latter is that they have limited degrees of freedom, which make some complex surgical maneuvers difficult to be accomplished [18].

Thanks to robotic technology, laparoscopy can offer equivalent wrist motion and three-dimensional vision as open surgery. However, although haptic technology has evolved a lot in the last 10 years, it is still in its early stages. Besides, this is still unclear how to certify haptic feedback as completely safe and stable. The main difference between handheld surgical devices, including mechanical instruments and some of the robotic-driven instruments, and telemanipulated surgical systems such as da Vinci is that handheld devices provide haptic feedback during the surgical performance. For instance, in suturing, haptic feedback offers fundamental information about the tension during the knot tying [24]. There are some laparoscopic devices in the market, for example the OptiGrip® grasper, that provide innovative solutions to deal with this lack of this haptic sense in minimally invasive surgery.

The learning curve is another crucial aspect when new surgical instruments are introduced in the field of surgery. In this regard, experienced surgeons have a tendency to obtain better results in surgical performance with a traditional surgical instrument [24]. This fact can be explained because expert surgeons have more experience with the classic instruments, which takes longer to learn new gestures and maneuvers for the new devices. For instance, during suturing tasks, experienced surgeons usually have a tendency to use the rotation of the forearm, even if the surgical instrument includes some kind of rotation mechanism [24]. Results from a retrospective study suggested that proficiency in LESS myomectomy using the RealHand® or the Laparo-Angle® (for suturing) is achieved after about 45 operations [42]. Therefore, the introduction of new handheld devices in surgery may require a training period in order to reach the appropriate level of surgical competence.

Many of the presented handheld instruments for minimally invasive surgery are still in early stages of development. Further efforts should be done in order to improve their functionality and make them more institutive and easy to use. A consensus on basic principles that make surgical instruments versatile and easy to use should be established. Ergonomic guidelines on the instrument handle design have been previously described by several studies [43–45]. Besides, innovative solutions to exploit the full potential of LESS surgery and address some of their technical limitation for surgeons should be explored.

6. Conclusions

In this chapter, we have reviewed some of the most extended handheld devices available in the market and described in the scientific literature for laparoscopy and LESS surgery. These devices seek to increase the surgeon's dexterity, precision, and ergonomics. They allow for easier access to otherwise difficult intracorporeal areas and improved instrument triangulation, thereby reducing the risk of potential mistakes and complications, which may also result in a reduced hospital stay. These handheld devices use different technologies, some purely mechanical and some other based on robotics or mechatronics technology. Mechanical devices are in general cheaper and easier to develop, so most of the available handheld instruments fall into this category. Regarding the instrument design, it seems that instrument handles with finger-operated joystick are more ergonomic and easier to use than a wrist control, providing similar surgical performance. Studies showed that handheld articulating devices facilitate intracorporeal suturing with similar surgery time and outcomes to conventional laparoscopy. Many of the presented handheld instruments are still in early stages of development. Additional efforts should be done in order to improve their functionalities and make them more intuitive. Besides, further innovative solutions should be explored in order to exploit the full potential of LESS surgery. The introduction of novel handheld devices in MIS should be accompanied by a comprehensive training period in order to reach the appropriate level of surgical proficiency.

Author details

Francisco M. Sánchez-Margallo[1]*, Juan A. Sánchez-Margallo[1] and Amir Szold[2]

*Address all correspondence to: msanchez@ccmijesususon.com

1 Jesús Usón Minimally Invasive Surgery Centre, Cáceres, Spain

2 Assia Medical Group, Tel Aviv, Israel

References

[1] Janki S, Mulder EEAP, IJzermans JNM, Tran TCK. Ergonomics in the operating room. Surgical Endoscopy. 2017;**31**:2457-2466

[2] Sánchez-Margallo FM, Sánchez-Margallo JA. Ergonomics in laparoscopic surgery. In: Laparoscopic Surgery. Rijeka: InTech; 2017. pp. 105-123

[3] Szeto GP, Cheng SW, Poon JT, Ting AC, Tsang RC, Ho P. Surgeons' static posture and movement repetitions in open and laparoscopic surgery. The Journal of Surgical Research. 2012;**172**:e19-e31

[4] Pérez-Duarte FJ, Lucas-Hernández M, Matos-Azevedo A, Sánchez-Margallo JA, Díaz-Güemes I, Sánchez-Margallo FM. Objective analysis of surgeons' ergonomy during laparoendoscopic single-site surgery through the use of surface electromyography and a motion capture data glove. Surgical Endoscopy. 2014;**28**:1314-1320

[5] Anderson PL, Lathrop RA, Webster RJ III. Robot-like dexterity without computers and motors: A review of hand-held laparoscopic instruments with wrist-like tip articulation. Expert Review of Medical Devices. 2016;**13**:661-672

[6] Fan C, Dodou D, Breedveld P. Review of manual control methods for handheld maneuverable instruments. Minimally Invasive Therapy & Allied Technologies. 2013;**22**:127-135

[7] Torres Bermudez JR, Buess G, Waseda M, Gacek I, Becerra Garcia F, Manukyan GA, Inaki N, Inaky N. Laparoscopic intracorporal colorectal sutured anastomosis using the radius surgical system in a phantom model. Surgical Endoscopy. 2009;**23**:1624-1632

[8] Ishikawa N, Watanabe G, Inaki N, Moriyama H, Shimada M, Kawaguchi M. The da Vinci surgical system versus the radius surgical system. Surgical Science. 2012;**3**:358-361

[9] Shibao K, Higure A, Yamaguchi K. Laparoendoscopic single-site common bile duct exploration using the manual manipulator. Surgical Endoscopy. 2013;**27**:3009-3015

[10] Ishikawa N, Kawaguchi M, Shimizu S, Matsunoki A, Inaki N, Watanabe G. Single-incision laparoscopic hernioplasty with the assistance of the radius surgical system. Surgical Endoscopy. 2010;**24**:730-731

[11] Frede T, Hammady A, Klein J, Teber D, Inaki N, Waseda M, Buess G, Rassweiler J. The radius surgical system—A new device for complex minimally invasive procedures in urology? European Urology. 2007;**51**(4):1015-1022

[12] Zdichavsky M, Krautwald M, Meile T, Wichmann D, Lange J, Königsrainer A, Schurr MO. Single-port live donor nephrectomy using a novel curved radius R2 surgical system in an in vivo model. Minimally Invasive Therapy & Allied Technologies. 2015;**24**:63-67

[13] Awtar S, Trutna TT, Nielsen JM, Abani R, Geiger J. FlexDexTM: A minimally invasive surgical tool with enhanced dexterity and intuitive control. Journal of Medical Devices. 2010;**4**:35003

[14] Criss CN, Ralls MW, Johnson KN, Awtar S, Jarboe MD, Geiger JD. A novel intuitively controlled articulating instrument for reoperative foregut surgery: A case report. Journal of Laparoendoscopic & Advanced Surgical Techniques. 2017;**27**:983-986

[15] Yoshiki N. Single-incision laparoscopic myomectomy: A review of the literature and available evidence. Gynecology and Minimally Invasive Therapy. 2016;**5**:54-63

[16] Dhumane PW, Diana M, Leroy J, Marescaux J. Minimally invasive single-site surgery for the digestive system: A technological review. Journal of Minimal Access Surgery. 2011;**7**:40-51

[17] Rettenmaier MA, Lopez K, Graham CL, Brown JV, John CR, Micha JP, Goldstein BH. Realhand high dexterity instruments for the treatment of stage I uterine malignancy. JSLS. 2009;**13**:27-31

[18] Jeong CW, Kim SH, Kim HT, Jeong SJ, Hong SK, Byun S-S, Lee SE. Insufficient joint forces of first-generation articulating instruments for laparoendoscopic single-site surgery. Surgical Innovation. 2013;**20**:466-470

[19] Cianchi F, Staderini F, Badii B. Single-incision laparoscopic colectomy: A new era in the treatment of colorectal cancer? In: Khan J, editor. Colorectal Cancer-Surgery, Diagnostics and Treatment. Rijeka: InTech; 2014

[20] Schips L, Berardinelli F, Neri F, Tamburro FR, Cindolo L. Laparoendoscopic single-site partial nephrectomy without ischemia for very small, exophytic renal masses: Surgical details and functional outcomes. European Urology. 2013;**63**(4):759-765

[21] Wendt D, Thielmann M, Melzer A, Benedik J, Droc I, Tsagakis K, Dohle DS, Jakob H, Abele JE. The past, present and future of minimally invasive therapy in endovascular

interventions: A review and speculative outlook. Minimally Invasive Therapy & Allied Technologies. 2013;**22**:242-253

[22] Kim SK, Lee JH, Lee JR, Suh CS, Kim SH. Laparoendoscopic single-site myomectomy versus conventional laparoscopic myomectomy: A comparison of surgical outcomes. Journal of Minimally Invasive Gynecology. 2014;**21**:775-781

[23] Sánchez-Margallo JA, Sánchez-Margallo FM. Initial experience using a robotic-driven laparoscopic needle holder with ergonomic handle: Assessment of surgeons' task performance and ergonomics. International Journal of Computer Assisted Radiology and Surgery. 2017;**12**:2069-2077

[24] Bensignor T, Morel G, Reversat D, Fuks D, Gayet B. Evaluation of the effect of a laparoscopic robotized needle holder on ergonomics and skills. Surgical Endoscopy. 2016;**30**: 446-454

[25] Sánchez-Margallo FM, Pérez-Duarte FJ, Sánchez-Margallo JA, Lucas-Hernández M, Matos-Azevedo AM, Díaz-Güemes I. Application of a motion capture data glove for hand and wrist ergonomic analysis during laparoscopy. Minimally Invasive Therapy & Allied Technologies. 2014;**23**:350-356

[26] Herman B, Zahraee AH, Szewczyk J, Morel G, Bourdin C, Vercher J-L, Gayet B. Ergonomic and gesture performance of robotized instruments for laparoscopic surgery. IEEE/RSJ International Conference on Intelligent Robots and Systems. 2011;**2011**:1333-1338

[27] Aykan S, Akin Y, Pelit ES, Gulmez H, Tuken M, Colakerol A, Semercioz A, Muslumanoglu AY. Impact of motorized articulating laparoscopic devices with three-dimension visualizing system: A pilot study. Journal of Endourology. 2017;**31**:174-179

[28] Sieber MA, Fellmann-Fischer B, Mueller M. Performance of Kymerax© precision-drive articulating surgical system compared to conventional laparoscopic instruments in a pelvitrainer model. Surgical Endoscopy. 2017;**31**:4298-4308

[29] Sánchez-Margallo FM, Sánchez-Margallo JA. Analysis of surgeons' muscle activity during the use of a handheld robotic instrument in laparoendoscopic single-site surgery. In: Duffy V, Lightner N, editors. Advances in Human Factors and Ergonomics in Healthcare. Cham: Springer; 2017. pp. 3-15

[30] Iacoponi S, Terán M, De Santiago J, Zapardiel I. Laparoscopic hysterectomy with a handheld robotic device in a case of uterine sarcoma. Taiwanese Journal of Obstetrics & Gynecology. 2015;**54**:84-85

[31] Sarlos D, Kots L, Stevanovic N, von Felten S, Schär G. Robotic compared with conventional laparoscopic hysterectomy: A randomized controlled trial. Obstetrics and Gynecology. 2012;**120**(3):604-611

[32] Pérez-Lanzac de Lorca A, Rosety Rodriguez J, Okhunov Z, Soto Villalva J, Garcia-Baquero R, Ledo Cepedo MJ, Madurga Patuel B, Alvarez-Ossorio Fernandez JL. Robot-assisted laparoendoscopic hybrid single-site radical prostatectomy: A novel technique using Kymerax. Journal of Endourology Part B, Videourology. 2013;**27**

[33] Trejo A, Jung MC, Oleynikov D, Hallbeck MS. Effect of handle design and target location on insertion and aim with a laparoscopic surgical tool. Applied Ergonomics. 2007;**38**(6): 745-753

[34] Rousek JB, Brown-Clerk B, Lowndes BR, Balogh BJ, Hallbeck MS. Optimizing integration of electrosurgical hand controls within a laparoscopic surgical tool. Minimally Invasive Therapy & Allied Technologies. 2012;**21**:222-233

[35] Leite M, Carvalho AF, Costa P, Pereira R, Moreira A, Rodrigues N, Laureano S, Correia-Pinto J, Vilaça JL, Leão P. Assessment of laparoscopic skills performance. Surgical Innovation. 2016;**23**:52-61

[36] Alleblas CCJ, Vleugels MPH, Coppus SFPJ, Nieboer TE. The effects of laparoscopic graspers with enhanced haptic feedback on applied forces: A randomized comparison with conventional graspers. Surgical Endoscopy. 2017;**31**:5411-5417

[37] Shang J, Noonan DP, Payne C, Clark J, Sodergren MH, Darzi A, Yang G-Z. An articulated universal joint based flexible access robot for minimally invasive surgery. In: 2011 IEEE International Conference on Robotics and Automation. IEEE; 2011. pp. 1147-1152

[38] Okken LM, Chmarra MK, Hiemstra E, Jansen FW, Dankelman J. Assessment of joystick and wrist control in hand-held articulated laparoscopic prototypes. Surgical Endoscopy. 2012;**26**:1977-1985

[39] Zahraee A, Paik J, Szewczyk J, Morel G. Toward the development of a hand-held surgical robot for laparoscopy. IEEE/ASME Transactions on Mechatronics. 2010;**15**(6):853-861

[40] Fan C, Clogenson H, Breedveld P, van den Dobbelsteen JJ, Dankelman J. Comparison of two control methods for minimally invasive surgical instruments. Journal of Medical Devices. 2012;**9**(1):75-82

[41] Santos BF, Reif TJ, Soper NJ, Hungness ES. Effect of training and instrument type on performance in single-incision laparoscopy: Results of a randomized comparison using a surgical simulator. Surgical Endoscopy. 2011;**25**:3798-3804

[42] Lee HJ, Kim JY, Kim SK, Lee JR, Suh CS, Kim SH. Learning curve analysis and surgical outcomes of single-port laparoscopic myomectomy. Journal of Minimally Invasive Gynecology. 2015;**22**:607e611

[43] Nesbakken R. Ergonomic guidelines in handle design - The challenges of laparoscopic surgical instruments. Student Project Report, NTNU. 2004. Available at: http://www.ivt.ntnu.no/ipd/forskning/artikler/2004.htm

[44] van Veelen MA, Snijders CJ, Leeuwen E, Goossens RHM, Kazemier G. Improvement of foot pedals used during surgery based on new ergonomic guidelines. Surgical Endoscopy. 2003;**17**:1086-1091

[45] van Det MJ, Meijerink WJHJ, Hoff C, Totté ER, Pierie JPEN. Optimal ergonomics for laparoscopic surgery in minimally invasive surgery suites: A review and guidelines. Surgical Endoscopy. 2009;**23**:1279-1285

Chapter 7

How to Prevent Irregular Adsorption of Fatty Tissue into the Irrigation-Suction Instrument

Tokihito Nishida and Hajime Ikuta

Additional information is available at the end of the chapter

http://dx.doi.org/10.5772/intechopen.76467

Abstract

Background: While using an irrigation-suction instrument for laparoscopic surgery, the irregular adsorption of fatty tissue may damage the tissue or obstruct continuous sucking. New devices of divided silicone drain tip and Count-on Q™ to prevent irregular adsorption of fatty tissue were reported. Materials and methods: A cigarette-type silicone drain was cut 4 cm in length, slipped over the instrument to cover the side holes, leaving 1.2 cm free from the end and fixed by means of 1-0 silk above the side holes. The free tip was divided vertically into four even pieces like octopus arms. Count-on Q™ was the irrigation-suction instrument equipped with multiple small side holes. Results: Divided silicon drain tip could prevent the irregular adsorption of fatty tissue (greater and lesser omentum or epiploic appendices) and could suck saline, fresh, and coagulated blood continuously. Count-on Q™ also could prevent the irregular adsorption of fatty tissue and could suck saline and fresh blood except coagulated blood continuously.

Conclusions: This simple, easy, and inexpensive device of divided silicon drain tip facilitated the prevention of irregular adsorption of fatty tissue while using a usual irrigation-suction instrument. Count-on Q™ was the masterpiece of irrigation-suction instrument, preventing irregular adsorption of fatty tissue by itself.

Keywords: laparoscopic surgery, irrigation-suction instrument, irregular adsorption of fatty tissue, divided silicone drain tip, count-on Q

1. Introduction

Several industrial companies manufactured irrigation-suction instruments that can be inserted into a 5-mm trocar for laparoscopic surgery. The instrument of 5 mm in diameter was equipped with a main end hole and 8–12 pieces of small side holes for 1-cm length of the end. However, when we used the instrument, irregular adsorption of fatty tissue, for example, greater omentum (**Figure 1**), lesser omentum, and epiploic appendices (**Figure 2**) into the end hole or side holes, was experienced frequently. The sucked fatty tissue should be detached with forceps (**Figure 3**), which might cause the fatty tissue injury or obstruction of continuous sucking. Bowel injury by such instrument during laparoscopic surgery was reported in 1995 [1]. Already in ophthalmology about silicone tip, a decrease in complications during cataract surgery with the use of a silicone-tipped irrigation/aspiration instrument was reported in 2005 [2]. A novel laparoscopic suction device for applying precise aspiration during laparoscopic surgery, sponge-tip suction tube, was reported to prevent suctioning intra-abdominal organs, such as the intestine and omentum in 2008 [3]. We firstly reported the details of a new device made up of a divided silicone drain tip attached to the end of an irrigation-suction instrument to prevent irregular adsorption of fatty tissue in 2015 [4]. Furthermore, novel endoscopic catheter for "Laparoscopy-Like" irrigation and suction inspired by natural orifice translumenal endoscopic surgery (NOTES) was reported to result in no mucosal injuries in the EIS suction in 2016 [5].

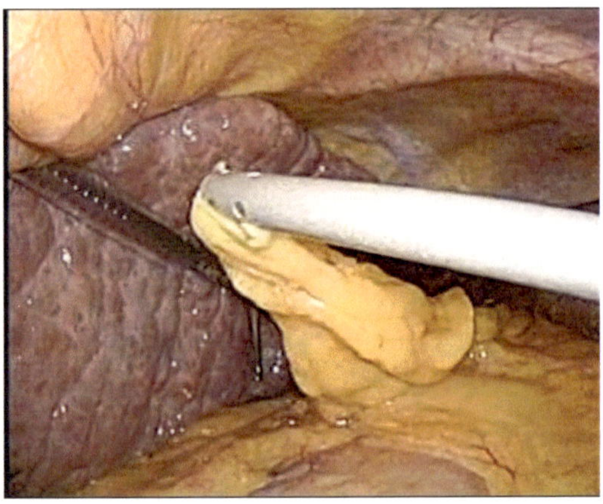

Figure 1. Irregular adsorption of greater omentum into a usual irrigation-suction instrument.

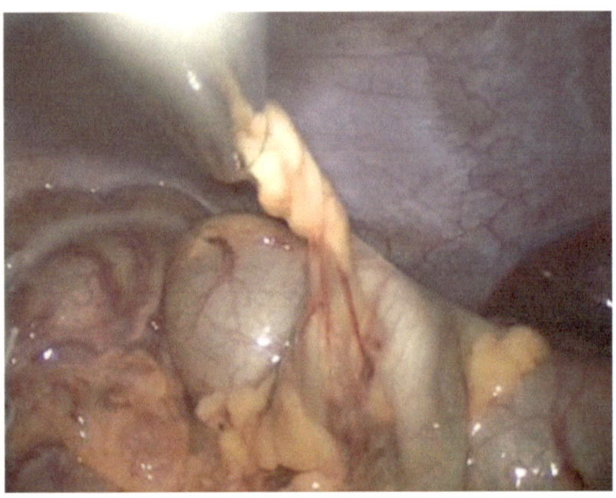

Figure 2. Irregular adsorption of epiploic appendices into a usual irrigation-suction instrument.

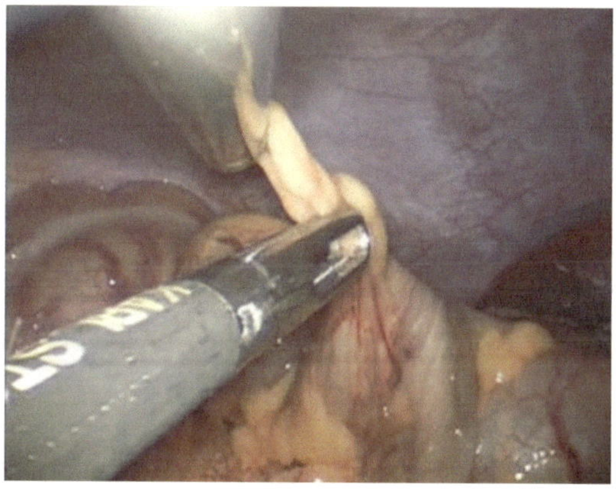

Figure 3. The sucked fatty tissue should be detached with forceps.

Herein, we mentioned the further experience of usefulness using divided silicone drain tip in several laparoscopic surgeries after the first report.

In addition, we mentioned another new instrument named Count-on Q™ (Pro-Seed Co., Tokyo, Japan), which was released in Japan in October 2014. This marvelous instrument could almost perfectly avoid irregular adsorption of fatty tissue by itself with multiple side holes while using it.

2. Divided silicone drain tip

2.1. Materials and methods

We previously reported the details of divided silicone drain tip (**Figures 4** and **5**) as follows: "We used a cigarette-type silicone drain of Type A No. 6 Penrose drain (Fuji Systems Inc., Tokyo, Japan). Type A means round, and No. 6 means 6 mm in outside diameter. The silicone drain was cut 4 cm in length, slipped over the instrument to cover the side holes, left 1.0–1.5 cm (1.2 cm was optimum) free from the end of the instrument and fixed by means of 1-0 silk at the central site above the side holes of the instrument. Finally, the free part of the silicone drain was divided vertically into four even pieces like octopus arms. As the instrument attached with the divided silicone drain tip could not be inserted from 5 mm trocar, it was inserted from 12 mm trocar or directly through the EZ Access (Multi channel port, Hakko Co., Ltd., Nagano, Japan) when placed on the abdomen [4]" After our first report in 2015, we used divided silicone drain tip for several laparoscopic surgeries of esophageal hiatal hernia, gastric cancer, colon cancer, rectal prolapse, appendicitis, liver cancer, cholecystolithiasis, and cholecystitis.

2.2. Results

An irrigation-suction instrument attached with the divided silicone tip could supply water straightly (**Figure 6**), which could avoid wetting the scope. The divided silicone drain tip could block and prevent the irregular adsorption of fatty tissue (**Figure 7**), and at the same time,

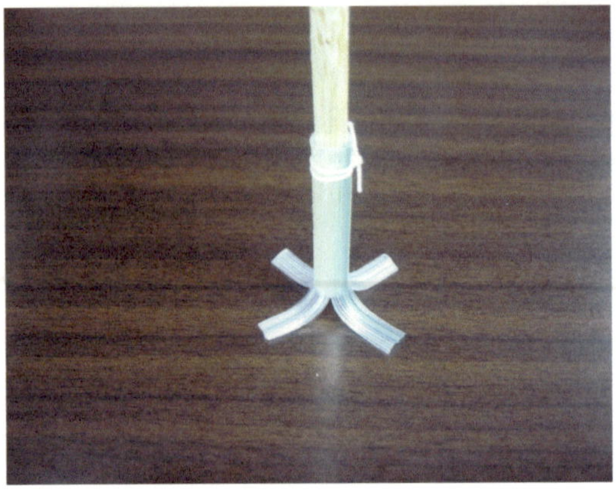

Figure 4. The shape of divided silicone drain tip into four pieces.

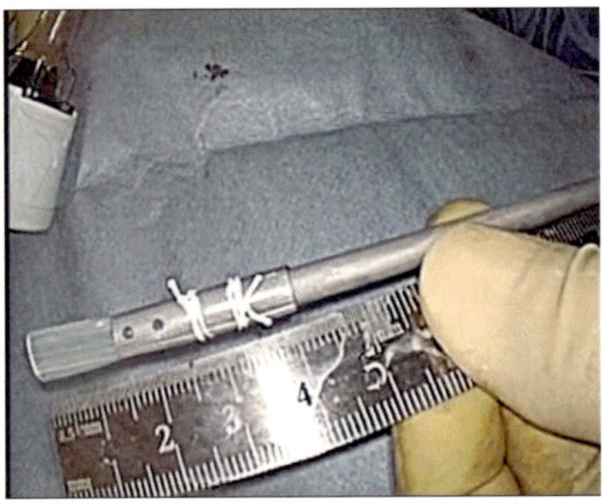

Figure 5. Silicone drain divided into four pieces at the tip of 1.2 cm was attached to a usual irrigation-suction instrument.

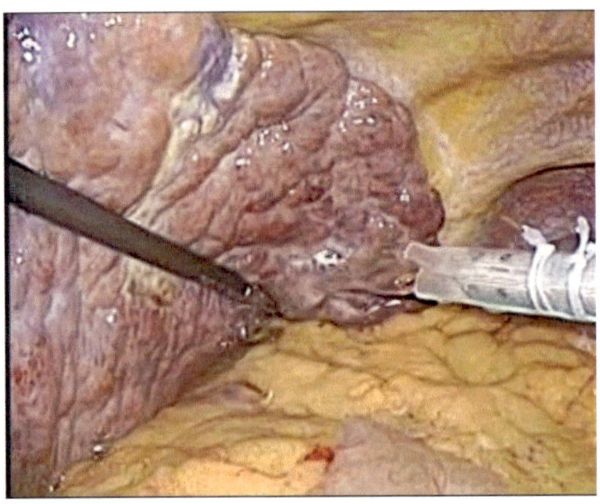

Figure 6. The divided silicone tip attached to an irrigation-suction instrument could supply water straightly.

saline or fresh blood could be sucked continuously (**Figure 8**). Coagulated blood also could be sucked through the divided silicone drain tip (**Figures 9** and **10**). This device would be effective for sucking a large amount of irrigated saline for a long time continuously.

2.3. Comments

As it was mentioned in the previous report [4], we studied reports on "irrigation-suction instrument" and "irregular adsorption of fatty tissue" in PubMed and Japanese Medical Abstracts Society Web (JMASWeb). There were no paper and only four proceedings of conference in JMASWeb (in Japanese). However, the technique was different from ours. We studied the optimum length and pieces of the divided arms in silicone drain tip. The length of 1.2 cm and the pieces of four were optimum. Silicon drain of 100% was flexible and had many fine vertical ditches at the inner side. These ditches enforced drainage and increased the tenacity of the arms to block fatty tissue. It could be detected with its X-ray impermeable marker when dropped in the abdominal cavity.

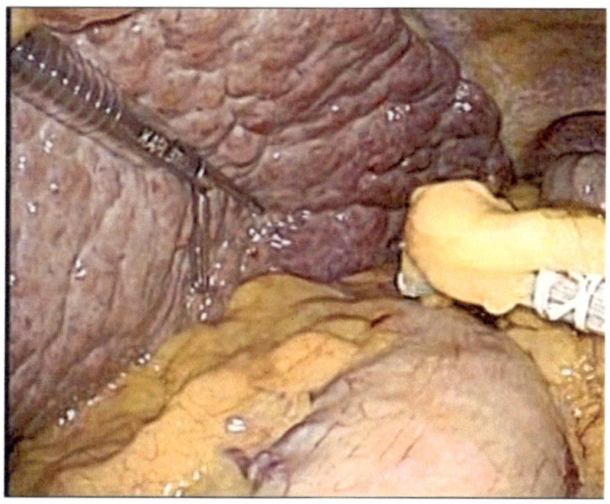

Figure 7. The divided silicone tip could block fatty tissue only to suck saline.

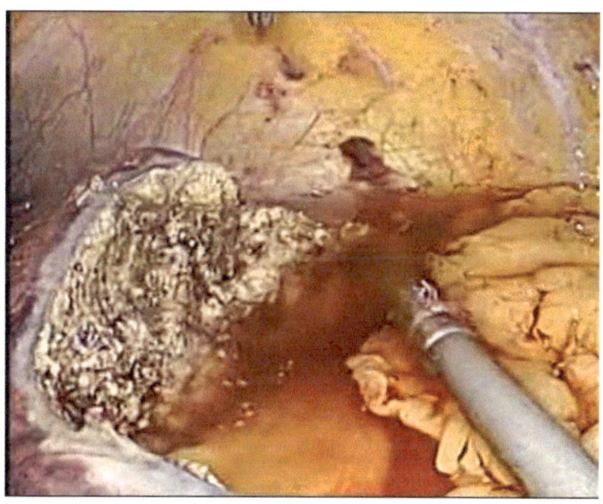

Figure 8. The divided silicone tip could suck saline continuously without irregular adsorption of fatty tissue.

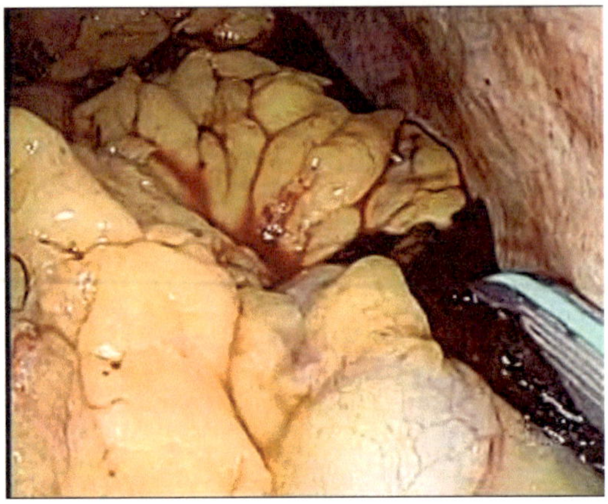

Figure 9. Before sucking the coagulated blood.

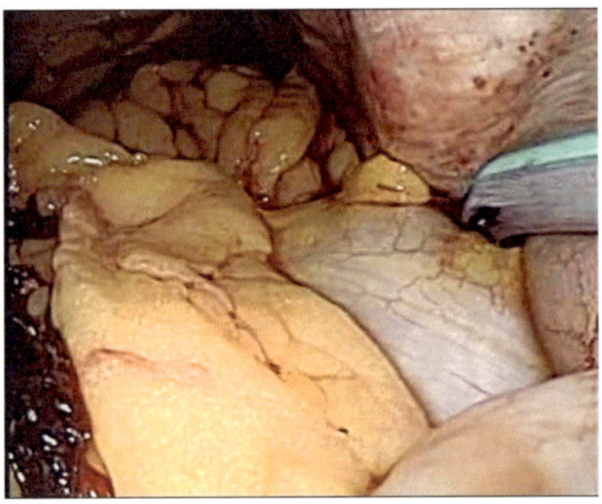

Figure 10. After sucking the coagulated blood.

3. Count-on Q™

3.1. Materials and methods

The Count-on Q™ (**Figure 11**), the basic concept that was devised by Dr. Atsushi Umemoto (Sainokuni Higashiomiya Medical Center, Saitama pref., Japan), was manufactured and released in Japan in October 2014. It was made of stainless steel, was re-usable, and had four types of lengths (32, 40, 50, and 60 cm). It consisted of an inner pipe of 4.0 mm in diameter and an outer sheath of 5.0 mm in diameter (**Figure 12**). The inner pipe was 0.5 cm shorter than the outer sheath, had a main end hole and four small side holes on the end and had a bulge of 1.0-cm length at the middle to seal the opening space from the outer sheath. The outer sheath

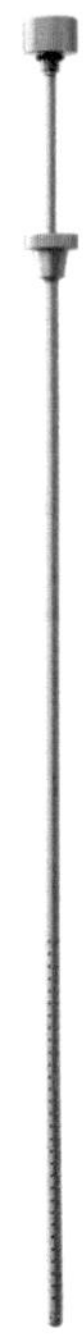

Figure 11. Count-on Q™.

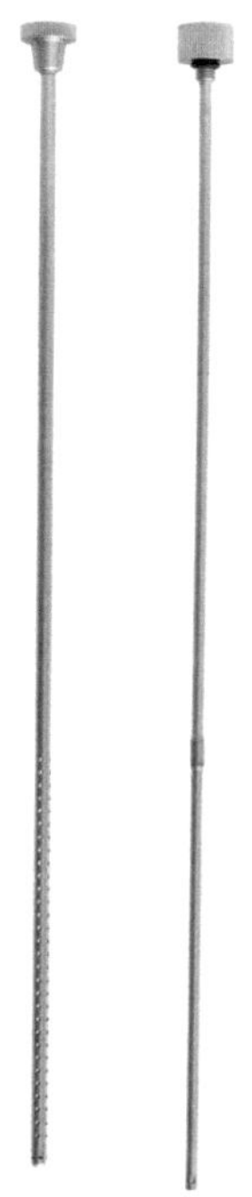

Figure 12. Count-on Q™ consisted of an inner pipe (right) and an outer sheath (left).

had five small holes on the end plane, four small holes on the end side, and 25 small side holes by five lines for 10.5-cm length from the tip (total 134 holes). Count-on Q™ was attached with a screw to the FineFlow™ irrigation-suction system (Pro-Seed Co., Tokyo, Japan) when using (**Figure 13**).

3.2. Results

We used Count-on Q™ two times in laparoscopic cholecystectomy and laparoscopic rectopexy for rectal prolapse. Saline was splashed in all directions (**Figure 14**) and could be sucked continuously without irregular adsorption of fatty tissue (**Figure 15**). Count-on Q™ could also suck fresh blood, but could not suck up the coagulated blood (**Figure 16**) and the small piece of tissue (**Figure 17**) because the holes were small. By the structural benefit, Count-on Q™ could suck only saline or fresh blood without sucking air while being sunk in at least 1-cm depth.

3.3. Comments

The same structural irrigation-suction instrument for open surgery had already existed. On the other hand, the concept to make the same one for laparoscopic surgery was marvelous. I tried to suck a cup of water by Count-on Q™ and could suck it up to the bottom of the cup without sucking air. In twice clinical use, we tried a large amount of irrigation and stress-free

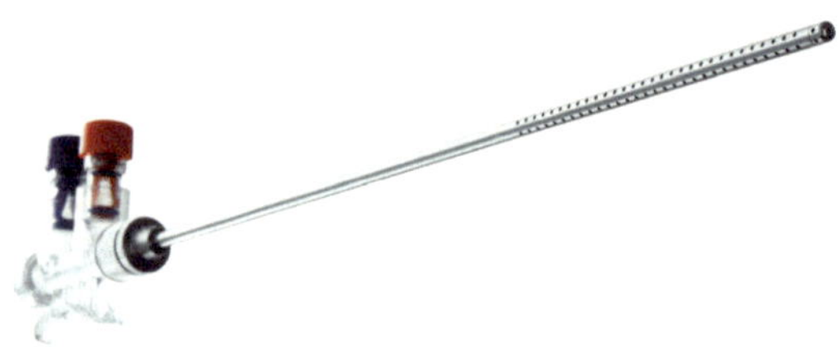

Figure 13. Count-on Q™ attached to FineFlow™ irrigation-suction system.

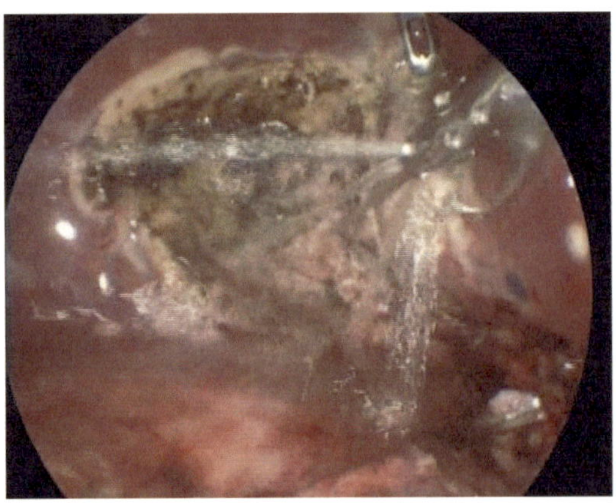

Figure 14. Saline splashed in all directions from count-on Q™.

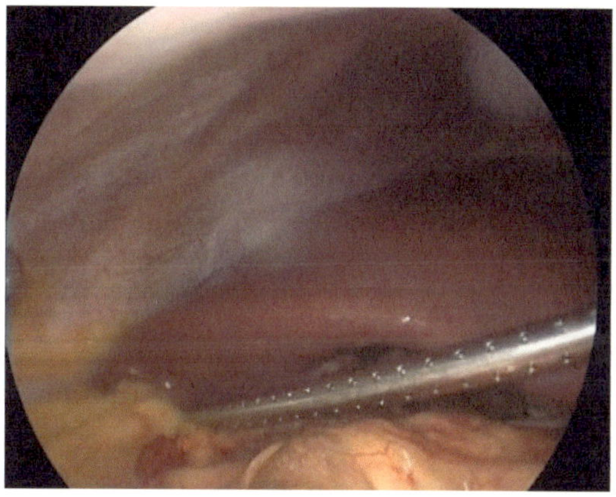

Figure 15. Count-on Q™ in the fatty tissue could suck continuously without irregular adsorption of fatty tissue.

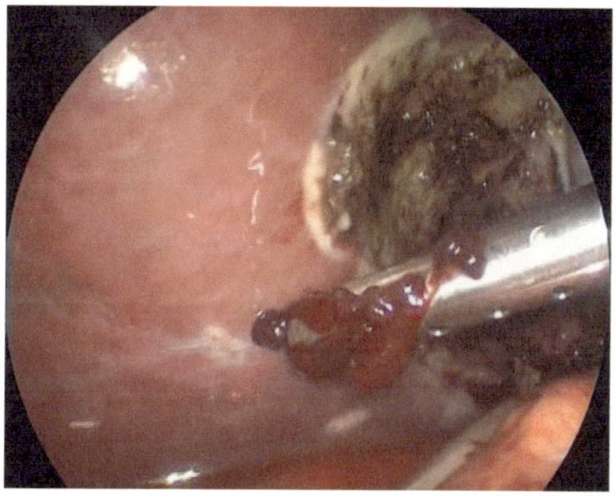

Figure 16. Count-on Q™ could not suck up the coagulated blood.

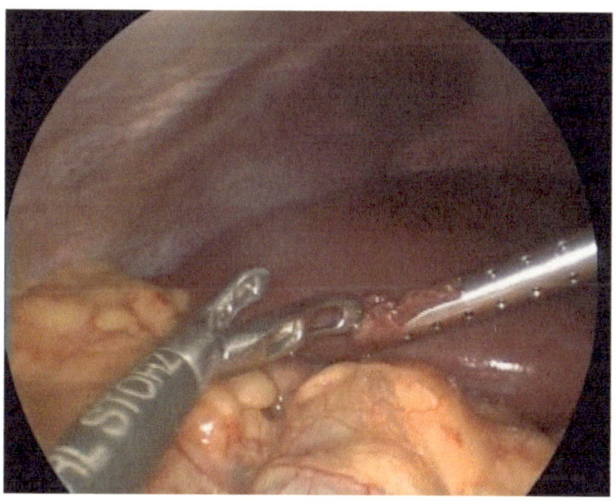

Figure 17. Count-on Q™ could not suck up the small piece of tissue.

continuous suction of saline and fresh blood. However, it could not suck the coagulated blood or the small piece of tissue because the holes were small. Therefore, it would be more suitable for a large amount of irrigation and suction for laparoscopic surgery of acute pan-peritonitis, for example, caused by digestive tract perforation.

4. Conclusions

Divided silicon drain tip was a simple, easy, and inexpensive device to facilitate the prevention of irregular adsorption of fatty tissue while using a usual irrigation-suction instrument for laparoscopic surgery.

Count-on Q™ was the masterpiece of irrigation-suction instrument, preventing the irregular adsorption of fatty tissue by itself.

Acknowledgements

I confirmed the permission from Fuji Systems Inc. (Tokyo, Japan) to use the silicon drain for this new method. I had no funding about this chapter.

Conflict of interest

I declare that there was no conflict of interest.

Notes/thanks/other declarations

I declared to express my thanks to Pro-Seed Co. (Tokyo, Japan) for the permission to report the Count-on Q™ with the FineFlow™ irrigation-suction system.

Author details

Tokihito Nishida* and Hajime Ikuta

*Address all correspondence to: tkhtnsd1957@yahoo.co.jp

Department of Surgery, Kasai City Hospital, Hyogo, Japan

References

[1] Wang CW, Lee CL, Soong YK. Bowel injury by the suction-irrigator during operative laparoscopy. The Journal of the American Association of Gynecologic Laparoscopists. 1995;**2**:353-354

[2] Blomquist PH, Pluenneke AC. Decrease in complications during cataract surgery with the use of a silicone-tipped irrigation/aspiration instrument. Journal of Cataract and Refractive Surgery. 2005;**31**:1194-1197

[3] MT1 O, Uzar AI, Eryilmaz M, et al. A novel laparoscopic suction device for applying precise aspiration during laparoscopic surgery: Sponge-tip suction tube. Journal of Laparoendoscopic & Advanced Surgical Techniques. Part A. 2008;**18**:747-750. DOI: 10.1089/lap.2008.0022

[4] Nishida T, Ikuta H, Yoshida S, et al. A new device to prevent irregular adsorption of fatty tissue while using an irrigation-suction instrument for laparoscopic surgery: Divided silicone drain tip. Surgical Laparoscopy, Endoscopy & Percutaneous Techniques. 2015;**25**:e104-e105

[5] Miyazaki Y, Nakajima K, Hosaka M, et al. A novel endoscopic catheter for "laparoscopy-like" irrigation and suction: Its research and development process and clinical evaluation. Journal of Laparoendoscopic & Advanced Surgical Techniques. Part A. 2016;**26**:943-949 Epub 2016 Jul 18